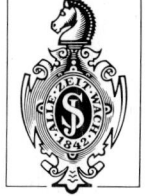

# Manuel Viamonte Jr.

# Errors in Chest Radiography

With 102 Figures in 296 Separate Illustrations

Springer-Verlag
Berlin  Heidelberg  New York
London  Paris  Tokyo
Hong Kong  Barcelona

Prof. Manuel Viamonte Jr., M.D., M.Sc.
Chairman and Director
Department of Radiology
Mount Sinai Medical Center
University of Miami School of Medicine
4300 Alton Road
Miami Beach, FL 33140
USA

ISBN 3-540-52906-3 Springer-Verlag Berlin Heidelberg New York
ISBN 0-387-52906-3 Springer-Verlag New York Berlin Heidelberg

Library of Congress Cataloging-in-Publication Data. Viamonte, Manuel, 1931–. Errors in
chest radiography / Manuel Viamonte Jr., p. cm.
ISBN 3-540-52906-3 (alk. paper).–ISBN 0-387-52906-3 (alk. paper)
1. Chest–Radiography. 2. Diagnostic errors. I. Title. [DNLM: 1. Diagnostic Errors–atlases. 2. Thoracic Radiography–atlases.    WF 17 V613e]   RC941.V46 1991   617.5'407572–
dc20   DNLM/DLC for Library of Congress    90-10322   CIP

© Springer-Verlag Berlin Heidelberg 1991
Printed in Germany

The use of registered names, trademarks, etc. in this publication does not imply, even in the
absence of a specific statement, that such names are exempt from the relevant protective laws
and regulations and therefore free for general use.

Product Liability: The publishers can give no guarantee for information about drug dosage
and application thereof contained in this book. In every individual case the respective user
must check its accuracy by consulting other pharmaceutical literature.

Reproduction of the figures: Gustav Dreher GmbH, W-7000 Stuttgart, FRG
Printing and bookbinding: Konrad Triltsch, Graphischer Betrieb, W-8700 Würzburg, FRG
21/3130-543210 – Printed on acid-free paper

# Contents

*Acknowledgements.* I am most grateful for the comments and constructive criticism made by Jack Cullinan of the Eastman Kodak Company and his wife, Angeline Cullinan, author of *Producing quality radiographs*. My thanks are also due to Peter Balanag, Head of our School of Radiologic Technology, for his valuable comments.

To my executive secretary, Peggy Litka, to my editorialist, Jan Holle, and to Lucy Kelley, program coordinator, my deepest appreciation.

# Introduction

Chest radiography is the most commonly performed diagnostic radiological examination in the United States. More than 80 million chest radiographs are performed annually in the United States and this type of radiograph accounts for 30%–50% of the total volume of diagnostic studies.

Standard chest radiographic examinations are difficult to optimize, primarily because of the seven- to tenfold greater attenuation of the mediastinum and heart than of the lungs. In order to obtain the best results, we must be able to see with distinct clarity the vascular markings of the lungs, particularly when these are superimposed on the rib cage, the bony structures, and the air–soft tissue interfaces of the mediastinum. The large variation in attenuation caused by the mediastinal structures cannot be recorded routinely on a radiograph with maximum image contrast. The lungs are shaped like a truncated cone. The apices are volumetrically smaller than the bases and are crisscrossed by bony structures (the upper ribs, clavicle, and sometimes the scapula and manubrium of sternum). Often in women, the density of the breasts overlaps the lung bases, and X-rays must therefore traverse more tissue.

Despite the cephalocaudal increase in tissue volume, it is possible in most instances to obtain a balanced density and contrast from the apices to the bases using the high kilovoltage peak (kVp) technique. Optimal image quality demands appropriate resolution and contrast that will permit the detection of pulmonary opacities and lucencies and of mediastinal and chest wall abnormalities.

*Resolution* is a measure of the sharpness of small anatomical structures and is characterized by the modulation transfer function (MTF), which is defined as line pairs per millimeter (lp/mm).

*Contrast* measures the difference in the attenuation of the X-ray beam which occurs between the bony structures and the soft tissues. It is influenced by object contrast (kVp and tissue attenuation coefficients) and scattered radiation.

# Technical Aspects

The proper technique for chest radiography requires that the high kVp technique be used and maximal contrast, spatial, and temporal resolutions be obtained. A high-powered generator – ideally three-phase –, which allows the use of high kVp (120–140 kVp), should be used. If a single-phase generator is used, the same penetrations are obtained with 147 kVp, as with 120 kVp, when using a three-phase generator. In addition to high kVp, ultrashort exposure allows detection of cardiac calcification as well as assessment of the pericardium. Ultrashort exposure is more advantageous for evaluating the heart than for studying the lungs.

The radiation dose absorbed by the patient is lower with the high kVp technique than with the lower kilovoltage range (80–90 kVp). Although high kVp reduces contrast, presenting a grayer image, the total information content from the lungs and the mediastinum is greatly improved.

This means better detection of parenchymal densities overlying bone in the lungs, and good delineation of trachea and proximal bronchi and of the mediastinal air-soft tissue interfaces.

## Film-Screen Combination

*Screen.* Absorption ability is the capacity of the screen to capture incident X-ray photons, and conversion efficiency is the ability of the screen to convert the captured photons into light. When we looked for the best screen, the rare-earth phosphor screens appeared to be superior to conventional calcium tungstate screens. High-speed calcium tungstate screens capture about 40% of the incident X-ray photons, but the rare-earth screens capture in the range of 60% of the incident X-ray photons. They also are more efficient in converting captured photons into light (5% vs. 18%, approximately). Because rare-earth intensifying screens admit the majority of their light in the green portion of the light spectrum, a special green-sensitive or orthochromatic film must be used in conjunction with these screens.

*Film.* Extended-latitude film should be employed. This allows proper exposure of the lungs and proper contrast of the mediastinal structures. With extended-latitude film, increasing exposure of the mediastinum still permits lung density to fall into an adequate and acceptable range.

## Techniques for Scatter Reduction

*Grids.* Scatter radiation is increased in the 100–140 kVp range. A 10:1 or 12:1 grid appears to be the most appropriate for this kVp range (a 12:1 grid at 140 kVp provides similar results to a 10:1 grid at 120 kVp). The airgap technique, where the patient is at a distance from the film, usually 10 feet ($\sim$ 3 m), and no grids are employed, is recommended by some authors.

*Fixed vs. Moveable Grids.* Some fine-line grids can be used as stationary ones. They will not produce grid lines that are objectionable. Many automatic changers use reciprocating grids. The use of a grid or a Bucky diaphragm improves contrast.

*Filtration of X-Ray Beams.* It is generally impossible to modify compensating filters for individual patients. Some manufacturers propose individual filters be used in given situations. Many people dismiss the use of these filters and believe that the high kVp technique and extended-latitude film suffice.

## Digital Radiography

Advantages over conventional film–screen systems can be achieved by using digital radiography. Among the advantages are the wider dynamic ranges allowing for unique contrast resolutions. It is also possible to have digital data immediately available for image transmission as well as multi-user display, manipulation, and archiving of images. On a theoretical basis, the radiation dose to which the patient is exposed can be potentially reduced by performing fewer repeat examinations. Therefore, for digital systems to be acceptable, they should first match the resolution provided by film–screen combinations. It has been stated that objects 1 mm in diameter require a spatial resolution of at least 2.5 lp/mm, a pixel size of 0.2 mm or smaller, and a contrast of 8–12 bits. Commercially available digital radiography systems do not yet match the overall resolution of the film–screen combination.

A second objection has been the high cost of digital technology. Despite the high cost of digital radiography systems, the quality of digitized images has improved to such a degree that we can predict that in time they may replace conventional film–screen combinations.

## Automated Chest Unit

*New Advances.* Automated chest units provide for phototimed exposure and produce consistent results. Most recently the advanced multiple-beam, equalization radiography (AMBER) system, in combination with the scanning equalization radiography (SER) technique, appears to be the best automated system for chest radiography. The SER system was developed by Plewes and colleagues at the University of Rochester. The AMBER system was developed by Odelft Company of the Netherlands. With these two systems the end result is uniform film exposure and improved image quality (contrast and resolution). These systems control the local exposure delivered to the film and use a slit technique to provide a fan-shaped X-ray beam which scans the patient vertically. The system consists of an X-ray source, filtrated by 1 mm Al and 0.5 mm Cu, and collimated through a front slit into a thick horizontal fan beam ($14'' \times 1.6''$). This radiation fan passes through a 20-channel harmonica-like aperture, where the height of each of the channels can be modulated from fully open (2 cm at the patient) to virtually closed (0.2 cm at the patient). The height of these apertures is continuously controlled by a feedback microprocessor. The patient's chest is scanned, from bottom to top in 0.8 s through a radiolucent set of 20 horizontally positioned detectors, which provide the micro-processor with the information needed to control the aperture heights, given the film speed and characteristic curve it has been designed to simulate. This horizon-tal linear array of detectors is itself protected by top and bottom lead-collimating panels, forming a rear slit.

The film–screen combination, either in a cassette or fixed chamber, is exposed in a focal-plane slit-shutter mode similar to some single lens reflex camera designs.

*The Beam Modulator.* Each beam segment has a modulator positioned in front of the X-ray tube and a detector between the Bucky diaphragm and the film cassette. The modulator uses absorbers on the tips of piezoelectric actuators as attenuation elements. Voltage to the actuators causes the attenuation element to bend, thereby partially or completely absorbing local radiation. Actuator voltage is controlled via a feedback loop from a corresponding detector, each of which is composed of eight xenon detector strips. The beam segments from the harmonica-like beam modulator move across the chest field at constant speed with straight, aligned front edges. The rear edge of each of the 20 channels closes in to reduce the area of irradiation at each moment of the exposure independently in each vertical track. This acts as a real-time exposure control mechanism, activated by the feedback signals from the detectors and processed by the microcomputer software, which simulates the sensitometric response of the film.

*Dosage Criteria.* The AMBER system initially aims for the exposure level needed to produce a chest image in which the mediastinum is ideally represented. In a conventional situation this would lead to blackened images of the lung field. To avoid this, the modulator locally modifies the beam segment size to make the average image density of the lung field areas similar to that of the mediastinum, enabling the diagnostician to see microstructures equally well in all regions. This approach suggests that only the dosage required for the mediastinum and diaphragm areas is slightly higher than when a conventional radiographic approach is used. In addition, however, most scatter radiation effects are eliminated due to the slit–scan design. This means that some film blackening attributed to scatter radiation has to be compensated for by modest increases in primary radiation. This overall dosage increase ranges between 5% for thin patients and 40% for heavy patients, according to Vlasbloem and Schultze Kool (1988) of the University Hospital of Leiden, The Netherlands. It is important to note that these calculations were done using a 400-speed film–screen system for both conventional and AMBER exposures.

Using this system, chest images are achieved with much more readily detectable fine structures in all areas. The lung images obtained with the AMBER system are the best achievable today, and the images of the mediastinum and retrocardiac space are significantly improved and match the lung image quality. Posterior and inferior portions of the lung, especially behind the diaphragm, can be visualized even in the PA view, a fact which will possibly affect the decision to order routine lateral views. Many chest examinations are today done on medium-speed rare-earth systems (speed 250). AMBER exposure protocols are set up for high-speed rare-earth systems (speed > 400). The potential to move to these higher-speed systems exists due to the strong signal content of the AMBER image-in-space.

Regarding new types of X-ray detectors, storage phosphor imaging is one of the most promising new techniques. It was first developed by the Fuji Corporation (computer radiography) and is now offered by Philips Medical Systems, Konica, Eastman Kodak, General Electric, and others. The storage phosphor system is expensive and connnecting this digital imaging method to a picture archiving and communication system (PACS) will cost even more.

Storage phosphor and equalization radiography appear to be the most promising and most developed methods.

## Summary

The requirements for optimal technique in chest radiography are:

1. Optimal technical aspects (see Table 1)
2. Optimal inspiration
3. Proper centering of the patient
4. Two views (occasionally supplemented by oblique or special views)

Table 1. Optimal technical aspects and conditions for chest radiography

| | |
|---|---|
| Generator | Three-phase, 1000 mA, 100 kW, 150 kVp |
| X-ray tube | 0.6 mm (10° target angle), 1.3 mm (12° angle), 10 000 rpm |
| Filtration of X-ray beam | 2.5 mm Al (0.5 mm inherent; 2 mm Al added) |
| Grid | 103 lines, (minimum); 10:1 or 12:1 |
| Intensifying screens | High speed, rare earth |
| Film | Medium speed |
| Processing | |
| Temperature | Adjusted to radiographic technique and film–screen combinaton |
| Replinisher rate | |
| Technique | Distance, 72"; 140 kVp; automatic exposure control |

# Errors in Chest Radiology

Errors in chest radiology are caused by improper technique, by failure to interpret results correctly, or by inadequate knowledge of the patients's clinical history on the part of the radiologist.

## Errors in Technique

Errors in technique include (a) under- or overexposure, (b) poor inspiratory effort, (c) off-centering (off-centering to a grid results in a severe unilateral grid cutoff), (d) rotation of patient, (e) the use of only one projection, and, (f) the presence of artifacts.

Proper indication for a chest study not only requires a correctly exposed radiograph but also requires that a lateral view be included. Specific areas of the lung are obscured by the diaphragm, the heart, and bony structures, and can only be visualized in the lateral chest radiograph. The lateral view also clarifies abnormalities noted in the frontal view, such as hilar versus juxtahilar disease.

We have observed pulmonary densities which were missed on overexposed frontal chest radiographs. Likewise, extensive involvement of the mediastinum with encasement of the trachea can be missed when dealing with underexposed radiographs. If the heart appears very white and the spine is not apparent behind the heart, the chest radiograph has been underexposed.

When the central X-ray beam is not centered and is aimed at one of the hemithoraces, the resultant iatrogenic hyperlucency can simulate pulmonary emphysema, massive embolism, or absence of soft tissues in the ipsilateral hemithorax.

Improper use of the film–screen combination and processing can also lead to errors from the presence of artifacts or from lack of representation of a pulmonary and/or mediastinal pathology. Improper positioning (rotation) of the patient can obscure certain regions of the lung, such as the hila, and can produce a distorted position of the trachea, which can be misinterpreted as a paratracheal mass. Poor inspiratory effort not only will lead to poor definition of the lower lobes, but also can simulate blunted costodiaphragmatic sulci, which are seen with pleural effusions and pseudocardiac enlargement.

According to John E. Cullinan, "the number one error by radiographers is the failure to use adequate contrast media (air) for the study. With automatic exposure equipment, variations in inspiration are compensated for by longer exposure times. With conventional timers, with less air in the lung, more exposure is required; as much as 2 to $2\frac{1}{2}$ times more MAs or an increase to 10 to 15 kVp. Radiographers using conventional exposure times soon learn to try for maximum inspiration. Radiographers using automatic exposure controls produce a variety of chest appearances (all proper densities) due to various degrees of inspiration".

## Errors in Interpretation

Failure to interpret results correctly are due to:

1. *Errors of omission.* Difficult areas to evaluate include the lung apices, juxtavertebral regions, peri- and retrocardiac regions, juxtadiaphragmatic areas, the hila, and cardiac calcification.
2. *Errors of commission (overreading).* Errors in evaluation include pseudoinfiltrates (crowded markings from hypoventilation), emphysema (overexposure, hypovolemia or off-centering of X-ray beam), and "chronic changes" (in the presence of senile lung and of interstitial edema).
3. *Inadequate clinical history.*

## Difficult Areas of Interpretation

Difficult areas to assess are:

1. Lung apices
2. Paravertebral regions, especially in upper thorax
3. Mediastinum
4. Juxtadiaphragmatic lung

Subtle pulmonary pathology may be obscured by small lung volume in the uppermost portion of the lung, the crisscrossing of ribs and clavicle, and often the presence of hypertrophic spurs at the medial sternoclavicular articulation. Whenever in doubt, obtaining of a frontal radiograph, with the patient's arms vertically stretched, or an apical lordotic view, is suggested. Pulmonary cancers have been confused with hypertrophic spurs. Pulmonary nodules have been diagnosed in patients with bone islands, an error which has then been subsequently detected by computed tomography (CT).

Centrally located masses may not be observed in the hilar or paratracheal regions, but may be noted below the tracheal bifurcation on penetrated chest radiographs. The only suggestion of a mediastinal mass may be displacement of the pleuroazygoesophageal line. Likewise, mediastinal abnormalities may be detected if displacement of normal air–soft tissue interfaces of the mediastinum, such as the posterior junction line, is observed. Minimal thickening of the right paratracheal stripe may not be appreciated unless a previous radiograph for comparative purposes exists. Pulmonary densities in the paravertebral regions may be totally missed on frontal radiographs, and on the lateral views of the chest they may not be seen or may be confused with hypertrophic spurs of the spine. Conversely, hypertrophic changes of the thoracic spine can be misinterpreted as pulmonary nodules.

There are definite limitations in the ability to recognize small pulmonary nodules. Standard tomography generally shows more nodules than standard chest radiography, and CT of the chest may even show nodules not detected by either chest radiography or standard tomography. In patients with soft tissue or bony sarcomas in which there is a high probability of pulmonary metastasis, chest CT is recommended prior to radical surgery.

The detection of hilar or juxtahilar pathology may be quite difficult. Occasionally, an increase in the density of hilar shadow may be the only indication of the presence of a hilar or juxtahilar mass. Lateral and/or 55° oblique tomography may then reveal the pathological process that would account for the increase in the density of the hilum.

It is imperative to compare results obtained at different dates. A sudden increase in the cardiomediastinal shadow may be the only sign of an extensive infiltrating tumor of the mediastinum. This abnormality may not become apparent unless a previous study exists showing the cardiomediastinal shadow to be smaller. Esophageal and juxtaesophageal pathology may remain undetected on improperly exposed radiographs. Properly interpreted studies may reveal deviation of the trachea in the frontal and/or lateral projection, air in a dilated esophagus, a displaced pleuroazygoesophageal line, and a small or absent gastric bubble.

The nature of pleural effusion or of a pulmonary infiltrate may be suspected by observing associated mediastinal and/or subdiaphragmatic pathology, such as adenopathies and hepatic and/or splenic enlargement.

A chest radiographic examination may be absolutely negative for pathology, yet the patient may die a few minutes later from a massive myocardial infarction, or may have extensive meadiastinal tumor at autopsy. Areas of akinesis or hypokinesis can only be detected by fluoroscopy, with gated chest radiography, or by noninvasive and invasive imaging techniques. Considerable difficulty in breathing can be the result of diaphragmatic dysfunction. The latter may be observed by careful fluoroscopic examination of the diaphragm.

A systematic approach for the interpretation of the chest radiograph must include careful examination of the following:

| | |
|---|---|
| – *Lungs* | Compare the right and left pulmonary zones. Assess carefully the lung parenchyma at the site of crisscrossing of ribs and clavicles. |
| – *Hila* | Evaluate the density and morphology of the hila. |
| – *Mediastinum* | Assess the retrocardiac region. Evaluate the cardiomediastinal shadow. Study the trachea and major bronchi. Assess the air–soft tissue interfaces. |
| – *Diaphragm and juxtadiaphragmatic regions* | Decide if basilar densities represent pulmonary, pleural, diaphragmatic, or subdiaphragmatic pathology. |

| – *Skeletal structures* | Study the ribs, clavicles, scapulae, and spine. Evaluate the soft tissue. |
| – *Neck* | Compare the two sides and study the larynx and trachea. |
| – *Upper abdomen* | Analyze the liver, stomach, spleen, and gas pattern of the upper abdomen. |

Pertinent clinical findings may be essential for a correct interpretation of the radiological examination and should always be available.

The following techniques are to be recommended in addition to the chest radiographs:

The *esophagogram* is a useful examination when posterior mediastinal pathology are to be ruled out.

*Computed tomography (CT)* may reveal pulmonary nodules not seen on chest radiographs. This technique occasionally allows the nature of pulmonary nodules to be determined, and makes possible the early diagnosis of fibrosing alveolitis, emphysema, and bronchiectasis. CT is specific for the diagnosis of fatty masses and some cysts, and is the best imaging modality for evaluating the stages of bronchial carcinoma.

*Scintigraphy, ultrafast CT and magnetic resonance imaging (MRI)* are particularly suitable for evaluating diseases of the heart.

*Sonography* is the best modality for studying pathology of the heart and pericardium as well as for studying juxtacardiac, paravertebral, and pleural fluid collections.

*Angiography* is the only suitable method for assessing the coronary arteries and is of great value for examining the pulmonary circulation, the heart, the aorta, and the systemic and pulmonary veins.

*Ventilation/perfusion scans* are more sensitive than chest radiography in patients with pulmonary thromboembolism (PTE). The chest radiograph is negative in 30% of patients with PTE.

*Endoscopic biopsy* is most suitable for inner-third lung lesions. Lesions in other locations should be biopsied under fluoroscopic control. Anterior and middle mediastinal masses can be sampled using the suprasternal or the paraxyphoid approaches.

Don't procrastinate! Do not observe the growth of a cancer. The second best approach to prevention is to diagnose and treat a small lesion.

## Pitfalls of Improper Technique and of Interpretation

The number of pitfalls of improper technique and of interpretation encountered by trained radiologists increases logarithmically when radiographic interpretations are attempted by the nonradiologist.

A recent study compared errors noted in nonradiologists' reports with those of the gold standard (proper radiological interpretations). Errors of interpretation can be subdivided into errors of omission and commission. False positive (overreading errors) and false negative (omissions) were recorded. Categorically, on a false positive the nonradiologist reported an abnormality when the radiologist concluded that no abnormality was present. On a false negative the nonradiologist read the film as normal, whereas the radiologist recognized an abnormality. The clinical significance of these errors was then assessed. A primary error was one judged to be of significance, or of potential significance, for patient care (resulting in incorrect patient management). Secondary errors were considered those not affecting clinical decision making or patient prognosis.

Of 1200 chest radiographs, there were 143 reports with discrepancies between interpretations (11%). Of the discrepant reports, 82 were judged to be important (6%). There were 97 patients in whom errors of omission were made (i.e., failure by the nonradiologist to diagnose one or several of 18 conditions; see Table 2). Seventeen (1.2% of the total cases) discrepant reports involved primary errors of overreading on the part of the nonradiologist. Examples of overreading that could potentially affect patient care included reading a chronic process in the lungs as an acute change. The remaining disagreements in chest reports involved either false positive or false negative secondary errors not having any significant potential to affect patient care (61 patients).

**Table 2.** Errors of omission: failure of nonradiologist to recognize and abnormal condition on the basis of chest radiography

| Pathology | No. of Patients |
| --- | --- |
| Pulmonary infiltrate | 9 |
| Solitary, noncalcified pulmonary nodule | 4 |
| Juxtahilar mass | 4 |
| Paratracheal mass | 4 |
| Pulmonary cavity | 1 |
| Diffuse pulmonary emphysema | 11 |
| Diffuse interstitial pulmonary fibrosis | 1 |
| Enlarged thyroid | 4 |
| Large hiatal hernia | 4 |
| Moderate cardiomegaly | 10 |
| Left ventricular aneurysm | 1 |
| Calcified aortic valve | 16 |
| Heavily calcified coronary arteries | 7 |
| Pleural effusion | 1 |
| Cervical rib | 1 |
| Paget's disease of the clavicle | 1 |
| Wedged thoracic vertebral body | 9 |
| Probable blastic metastasis | 9 |
| Total | 97 |

The following were considered here to be unimportant findings:

- Degenerative changes of the spine
- Tortuous, dilated aorta
- Kyphoscoliosis
- Pectus carinatum
- Pectus excavatum
- Diffuse osteopenia
- Minimal loss of height of vertebrae in osteopenic individuals
- Old inflammatory changes in the lungs
- Elevated hemidiaphragm due to eventration
- Minimal calcification of carotid arteries
- Minimal cardiac enlargement
- Calcified pulmonary nodules
- Old rib fractures

Several patients had several radiographic abnormalities on studies the nonradiologist declared negative.

This study reaffirms the adage that "two heads are better than one," particularly when one head belongs to a trained, dedicated, and interested specialist.

# References

Aberle DR, Hansell D, Huang HK (1990) Current status of digital projection radiography of the chest. J Thorac Imaging Vol 5, No 1

American Cancer Society (1980) Guidelines for the cancer-related checkup. Recommendations and rationale. CA 30:191–240

Auerbach O, Garfinkel L, Parks V (1979) Scar cancer of the lung. Cancer 43:636–642

Austin J (1987) Missed bronchogenic carcinoma: potentially resectable lesions evident in retrospect on plain chest radiographs. Radiological Society of North America, Chicago, IL, 29 November 1987

Bakris G (1983) Pulmonary scar carcinoma: a clinicopathologic analysis. Cancer 52:493

Barnes GT (1988) Electronic imaging systems for chest radiography: an overview. In: Peppler WW, Alter A (eds) Proceedings of the chest imaging conference 1987. Medical Physics Publishing Corp, Madison, pp 178–193

Brogdon B (1983) Factors affecting perception of pulmonary lesions. Radiol Clin North Am 21:633–654

Castle JW (1977) Sensitivity of radiographic screens to scattered radiation and its relationship to image contrast. Radiology 122:805–809

Chahinian P (1972) Relationship between tumor doubling time and anatomoclinical features in 50 measurable pulmonary cancers. Chest 61:340–345

Cooperstein LA, Good BC, Eelkema EA, Sumkin JH, Tabor EK, Sidorovich K, Curtin HD, Yousem SA (1990) The effect of clinical history on chest radiograph interpretations in a PACS environment. Investigative Radiology 25 (6):670–674

Cullinan A (1987) Producing quality radiographs. Lippincott, Philadelphia

Don C (1988) The future of radiography–cassetteless or filmless? JK Can Assoc Radiol 39:83–90

Doubilet P, Herman PG (1981) Interpretation of radiographs: effect of clinical history. AJR 137:1055–1058

Fleischner F, Sachsse E (1963) Retrotracheal lymphadenopathy in bronchial carcinoma, revealed by the barium-filled esophagus. AJR 90:792

Forrest JV, Friedman PJ (1981) Radiologic errors in patients with lung cancer. West J Med 134:845–490

Frank MS (1990) New chest imaging methods for nodule detection and evaluation. Current Opinion Radiology 2:374–380

Fuhrman CR, Deutsch M, Gurd D et al. (1988) Digital radiography using storage phosphors. In: Chiesa A (ed) Proceedings of the fifth international symposium on the planning of radiological departments. Clas International, Brescia, pp 306–309

Fuhrman CR, Gur D, Good B et al. (1988) Storage phosphor radiographs vs conventional films: interpreters' perceptions of diagnostic quality. AJR 150:1011–1014

Fuhrman CR, Gurd D, Schaetzing R (1990) High resolution digital imaging with storage phosphorus. J Thorac Imaging Vol 5, No 1

Goodman LR, Wilson CR, Foley WD (1988) Digital radiography of the chest: promises and problems. AJR 150:1241–1252

Kogutt MS, Jones JP, Perkins DD (1988) Low-dose digital computed radiography in pediatric chest imaging. AJR 151:775–779

Lee MM, Wick MM (1990) Bowen's disease. CA-A Cancer Journal for Clinicians 40 (4):237–242

Merritt CRB (1988) Photostimulable phosphors – clinical results. In: Peppler WW, Alter A (eds) Proceedings of the chest imaging conference 1987. Medical Physics Publishing Corp, Madison, pp 208–211

Niklason LT, Sorenson JA, Nelson JA (1981) Scattered radiation in chest radiography. Med Phys 8:677–681

Plewes DB (1983) A scanning system for chest radiography with regional exposure control: theroretical considerations. Med Phys 10:646–654

Plewes DB, Vogelstein EE (1983) A scanning system for chest radiography with regional exposure control: practical implementation. Med Phys 10:655–663

Ravin CE (1988) Advanced multiple beam equalization radiography (AMBER): early clinical experience. In: Peppler WW, Alter A (eds) Proceedings of the chest imaging conference 1987. Medical Physics Publishing Corp, Madison, pp 60–63

Ravin CE, Johnson GA (1983) The optimal chest radiograph. 5:1–14

Rickert RR, Brodkin RH, Hulter RVP (1977) Bowen's disease. CA 27:160–166

Rickett RR, Brodkin RH, Hulter RVP (1977) Bowen's disease. CA-A Cancer Journal for Clinicians 27 (3):162–166

Sorenson JA, Niklason LT, Knutti DF (1980) Performance characteristics of improved antiscatter grids. Med Phys 7:525–528

Vlasbloem H, Schultze Kool LJ (1988) AMBER: a scanning multiple-beam equalization system for chest radiography. Radiology 169:29–34

Wandtke JC (1990) Newer imaging methods in chest radiography. J Thorac Imaging 5:1

Wandtke JC, Plewes DB (1985) Chest equalization radiography. J Thorac Imaging 1:14–20

Wandtke JC, Plewes DB (1989) Comparison of scanning equalization and conventional chest radiography. Radiology 172:641–645

# Atlas

## Figures 1–102

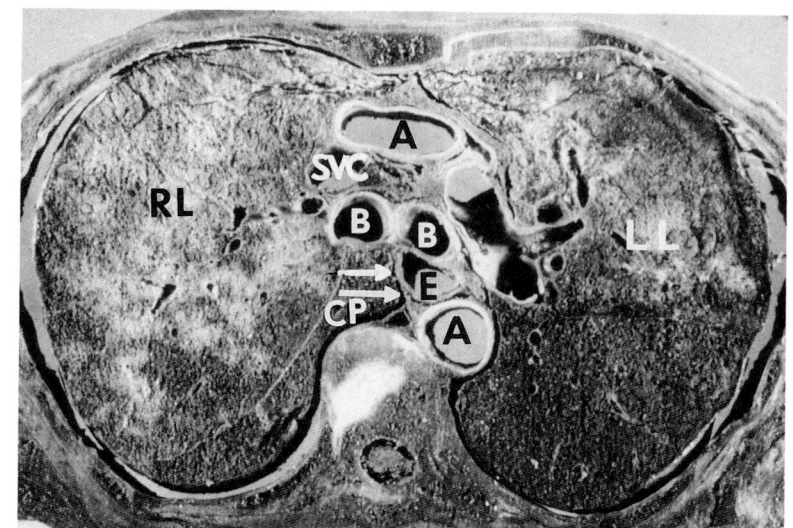

a

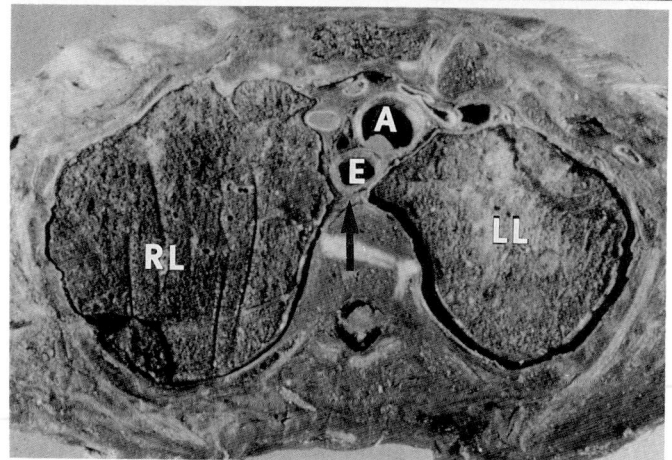

b

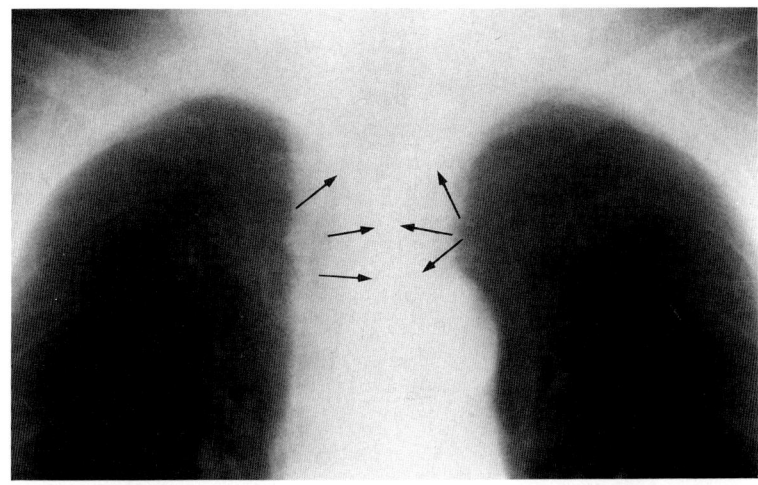

c

**Fig. 1a–c.** Air–soft tissue interfaces of the mediastinum (cadaver sections). **a** Pleuroazy-goesophageal line (*arrows*). *CP*, crista pulmonis (medial extension of right lower lobe); *A*, aorta; *E*, esophagus; *B*, bronchi; *SVC*, superior vena cava; *RL*, right lung; *LL*, left lung. **b** Posterior junction line (*arrow*); *E* esophagus; *A*, aorta; *RL*, right lung; *LL*, left lung. **c** Posterior junction line (*arrows*)

18

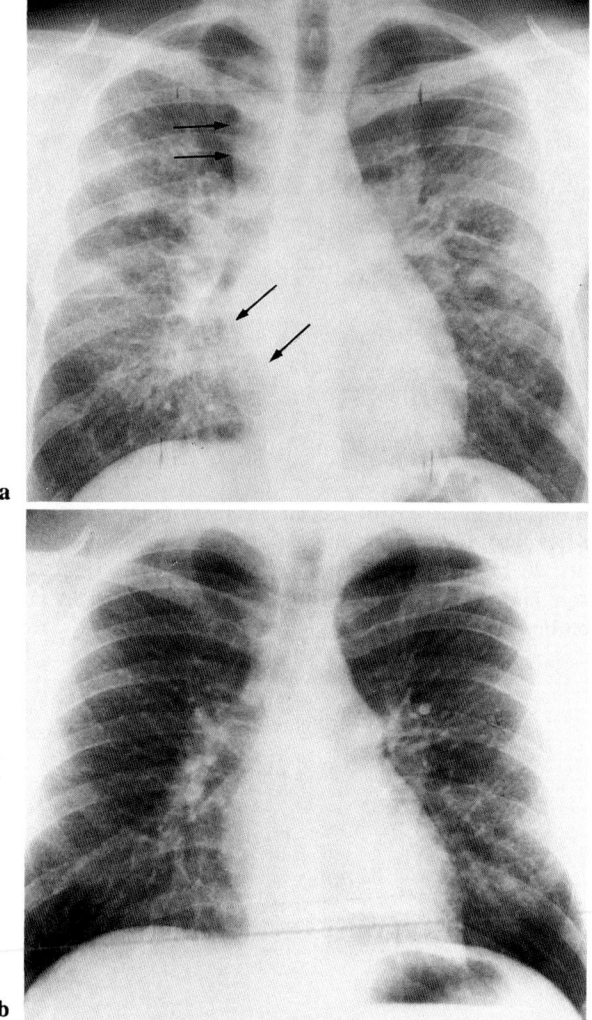

a

b

**Fig. 2a, b.** Importance of using the high kVp technique. Patient with sarcoidosis. a Note diffuse pulmonary infiltrates, right paratracheal mass (*horizontal arrows*), and displaced pleuroazygoesophgageal line simulating left atrial enlargement (*oblique arrows*). The patient had no evidence of cardiac disease. b Following treatment with corticosteroids the patient's condition returned to normal. The retrocardiac mass corresponded to subcarinal adenopathies. The pulmonary infiltrates with mediastinal involvement narrowed the differential diagnosis down to granulomatous disease and tumor

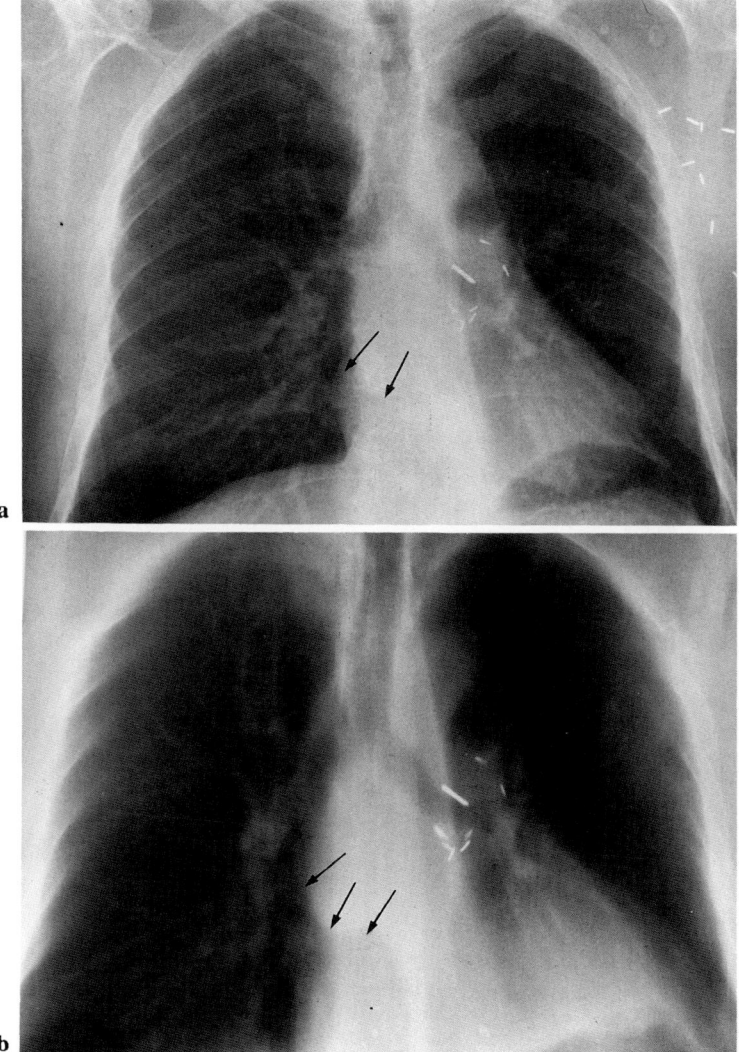

a

b

Fig. 3a, b. Importance of using the high kVp technique. Patient with melanoma. a Note displaced pleuroazygoesophageal line (*arrows*). There are surgical clips in the left hilum and in the soft tissues of the left axilla. Evidence of subcarinal adenopathies were the only abnormalities observed. b Linear tomography revealing to best advantage the subcarinal process, not manifested by a mass, but by simple displacement of a normal structure (*arrows*). At autopsy, extensive metastasis to the mediastinum were present

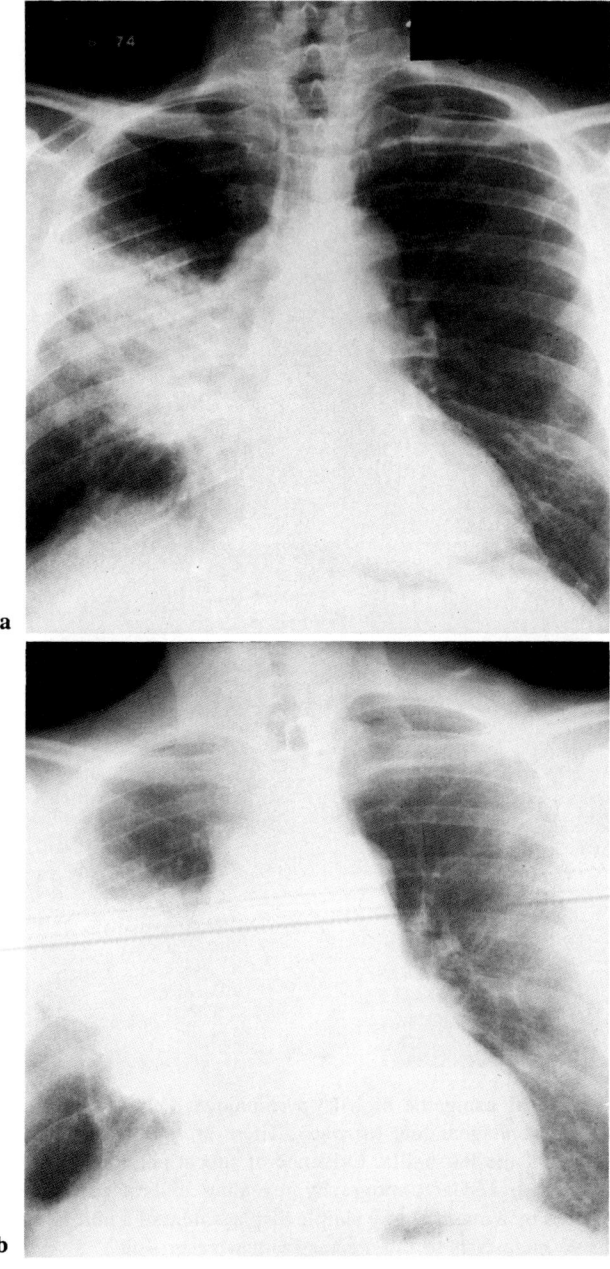

**Fig. 4a, b.** Importance of using the high kVp technique. Patient with Hodgkin's disease. **a** Note consolidation of the right lung with absence of the pleuroazygoesophageal line. The patient was treated for pneumonia. **b** Despite antibiotic treatment the pulmonary mass increased in size. At postmortem the mass was found to represent Hodgkin's disease. The fact that there was a mediastinal component should have led to revision of the diagnosis of pneumonia despite the presence of fever, cough, and chills which suggested an infectious process

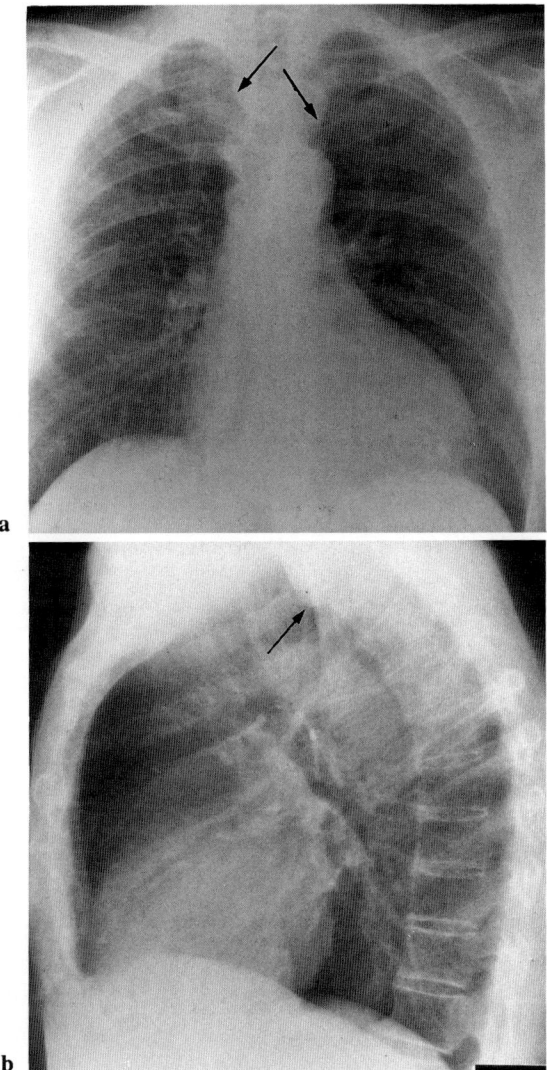

**Fig. 5a, b.** Importance of using the high kVp technique. Prevertebral monilial abscess.
**a** Frontal view only revealed at first glance enlargement of the heart and clear lungs. However,
the displacement of the posterior junction line caused by a supraaortic mass was barely
perceptible (*arrows*). **b** Lateral view of same patient. Note prevertebral process above aortic
arch (*arrow*). This proved to be a monilial abscess

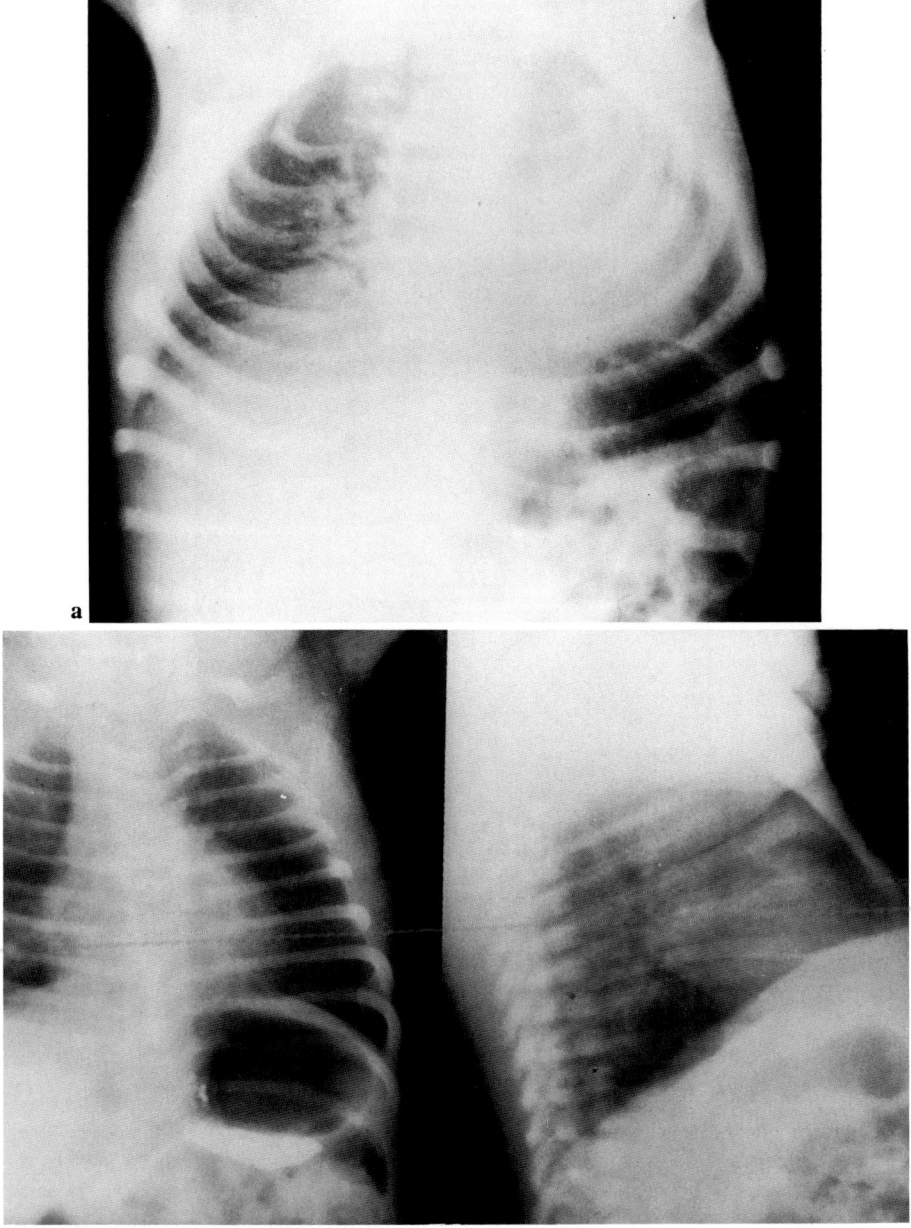

**Fig. 6a, b.** Importance of proper centering. **a** Bizarre appearance of the chest in a new-born. **b** Frontal (*left*) and lateral (*right*) views of the chest following proper centering. No abnormalities were present

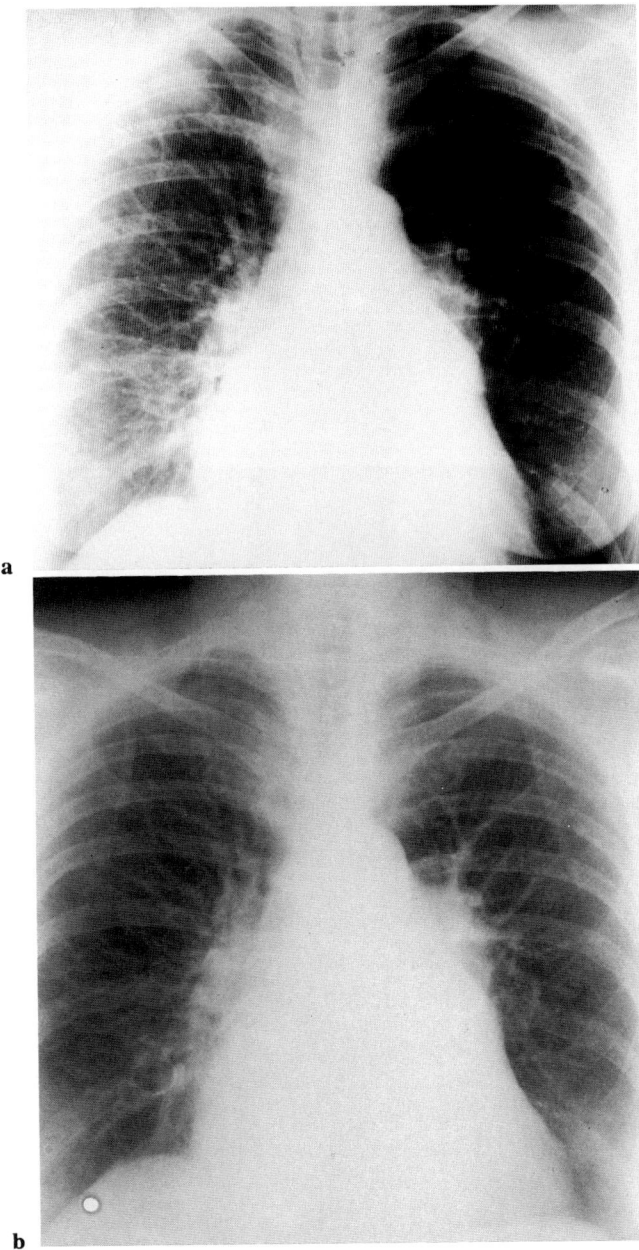

**Fig. 7a, b.** Importance of proper centering. **a** Patient not centered properly showing mitral stenosis and hyperlucent left lung. Differential diagnosis would include massive pulmonary embolization and emphysema. **b** Patient properly centered. Note equal aeration of the two lung. The iatrogenic hyperlucency observed previously was related to off-centering of the X-ray beam. The different density of the lateral rib cage, and shoulders is a clue to off-centering of the X-ray beam

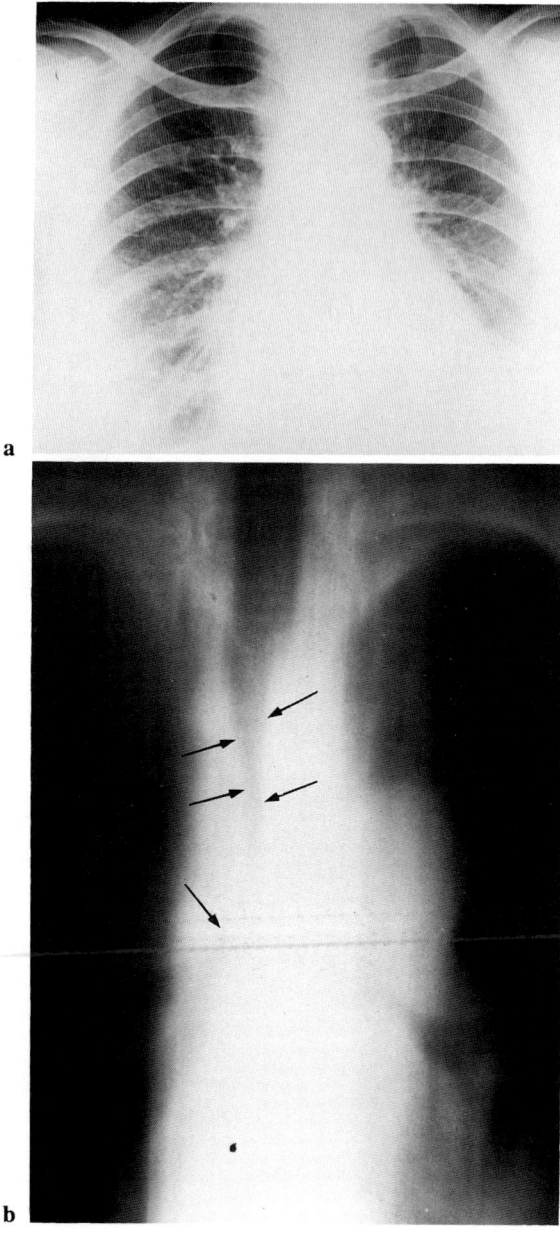

Fig. 8a, b. Underexposure. **a** Chest radiograph showed false abnormalities in the lung bases and poor definition of the mediastinum. **b** Linear tomography revealed diffuse encasement of the distal trachea and proximal bronchi due to mediastinal carcinoma. Due to the lack of penetration, the mediastinal abnormality was undetected in the underexposed film

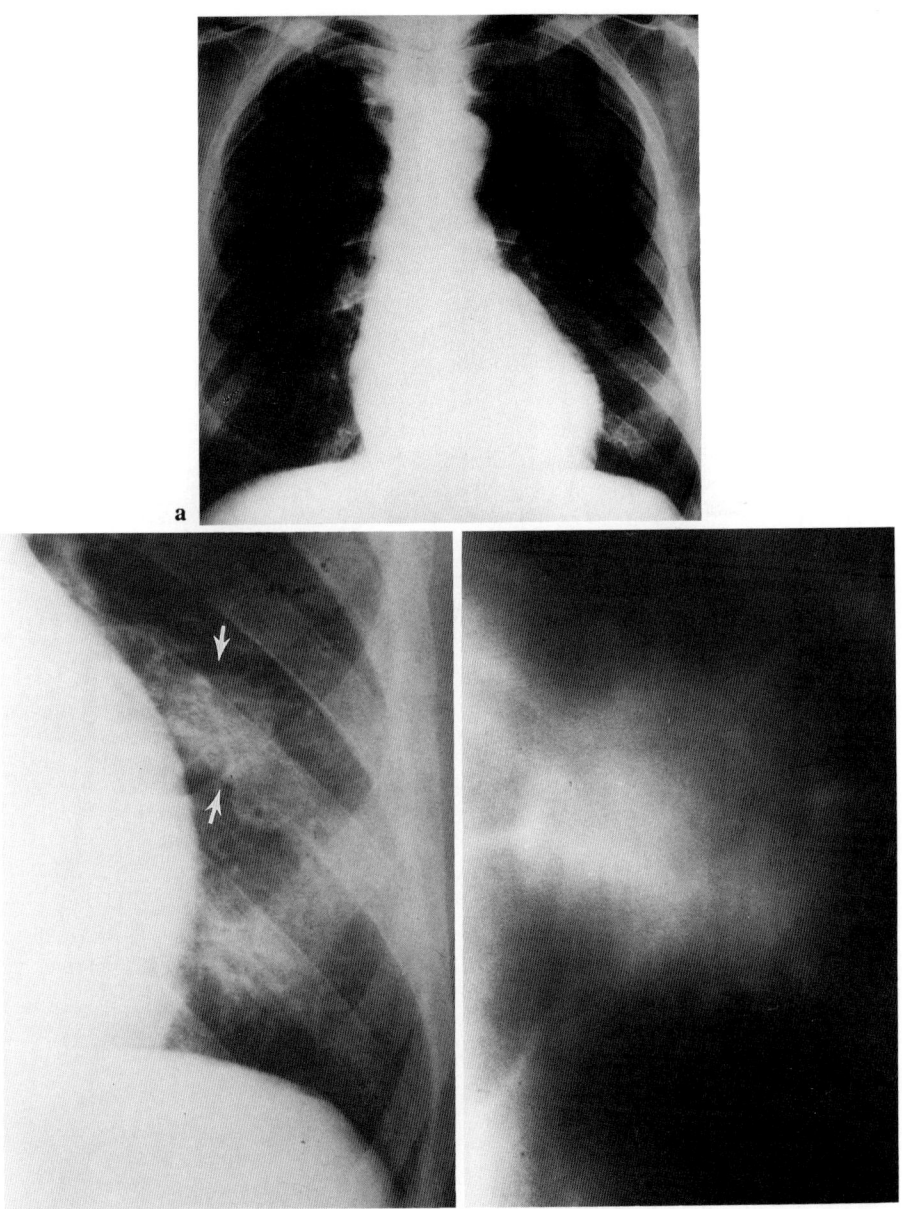

**Fig. 9a–c.** Overexposure. **a** The frontal view revealed very dark lungs. **b** When the left paracardiac region was lit brightly an infiltrate was noted (*arrows*). **c** A year later the patient returned with a nonresectable carcinoma

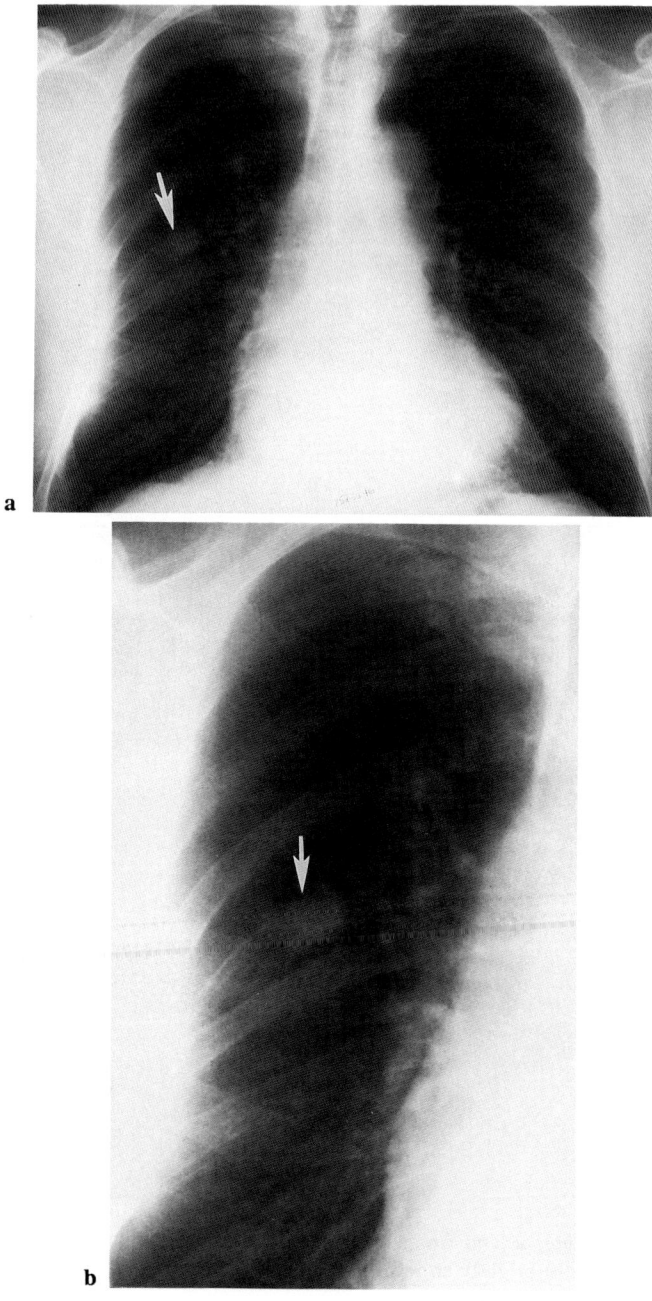

**Fig. 10a, b.** Overexposure. **a** The frontal view showed an ill-defined density in the right mid-lung field (*arrow*) which was overlooked. **b** A close-up of the right lung with transillumination showed an ill-defined nodule (*arrow*) which proved to be a bronchial carcinoma

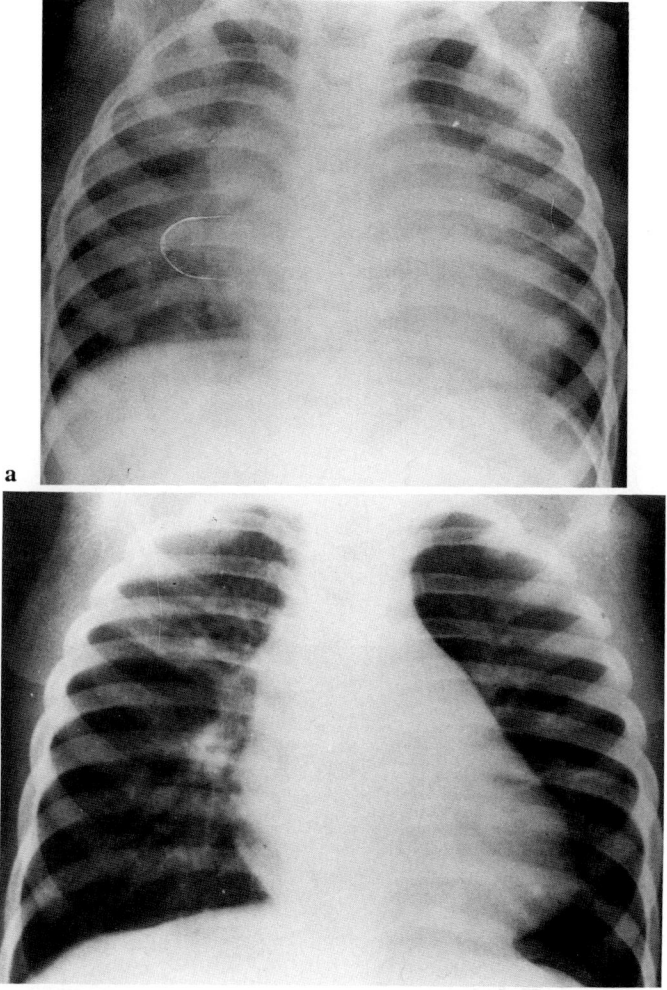

**Fig. 11a, b.** Effect of poor inspiratory effort. **a** Film of expiratory phase showing pseudoin-filtrates bilaterally and pseudocardiomegaly. **b** Good inspiratory phase. Note well-aerated lungs and a normal cardiomediastinal shadow

28

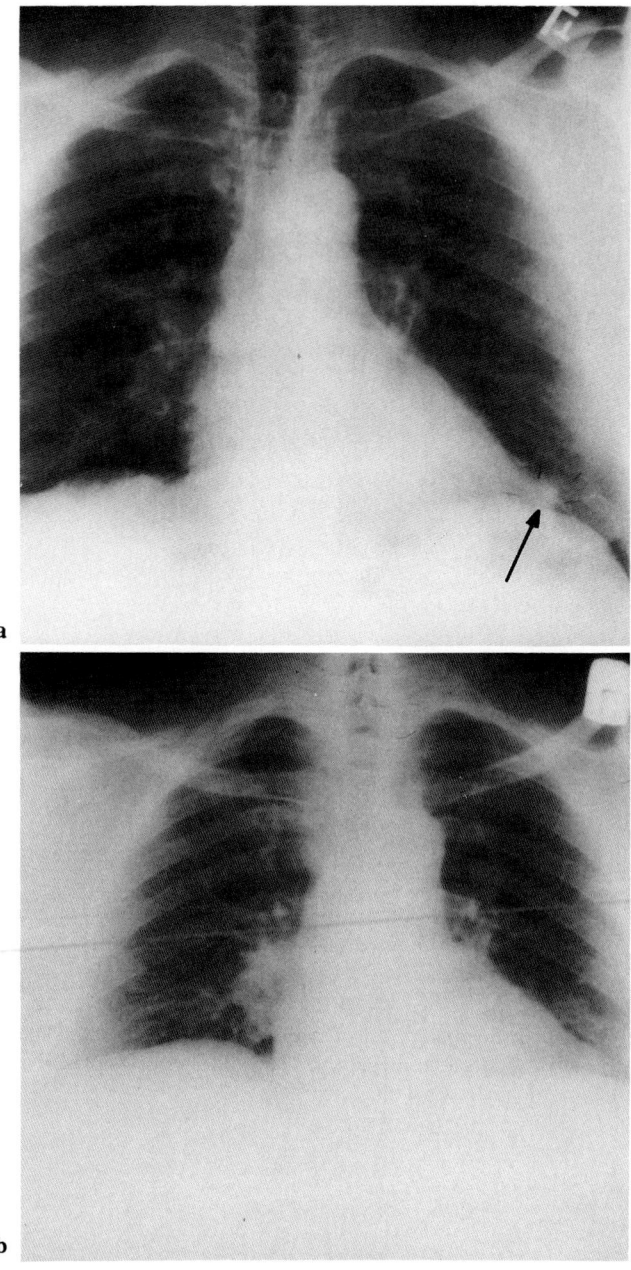

**Fig. 12a, b.** Effect of poor inspiratory effort. **a** Film of good inspiratory phase shows nodule adjacent to left cardiac apex (*arrow*) which proved to be a bronchogenic carcinoma. **b** Frontal view of the same patient in expiration. Nodule is not observed (obscured by diaphragm)

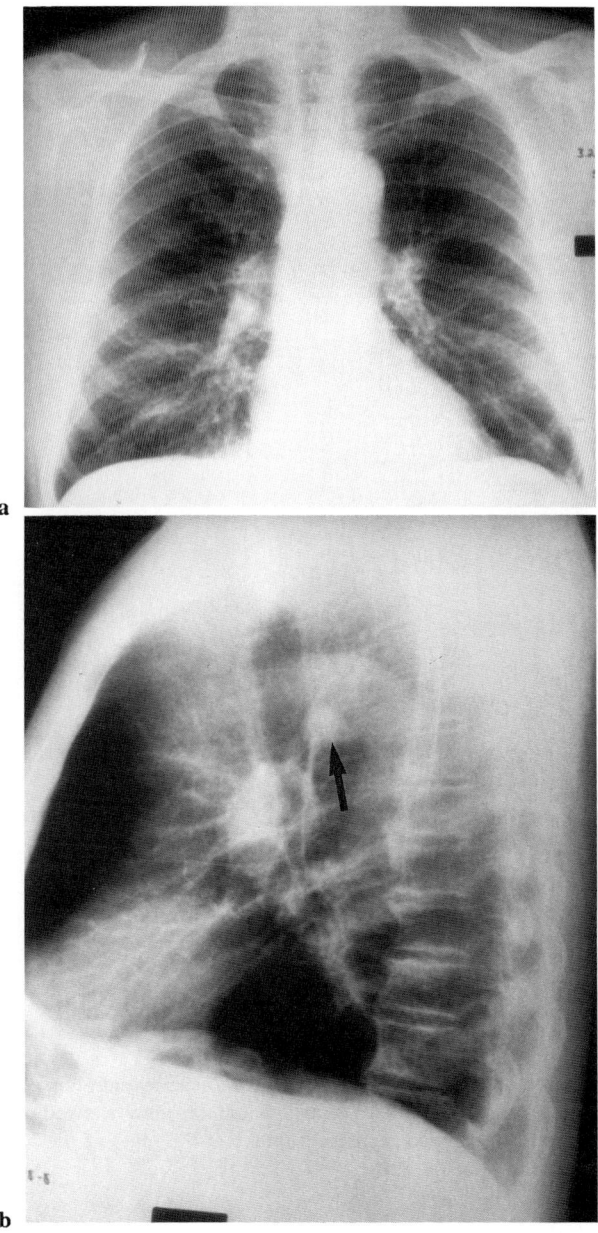

**Fig. 13a, b.** Importance of including a lateral view. **a** Negative frontal view chest radiograph. **b** Nodule below aortic arch (*arrow*) observed in lateral view radiograph proved to be a bronchial carcinoma

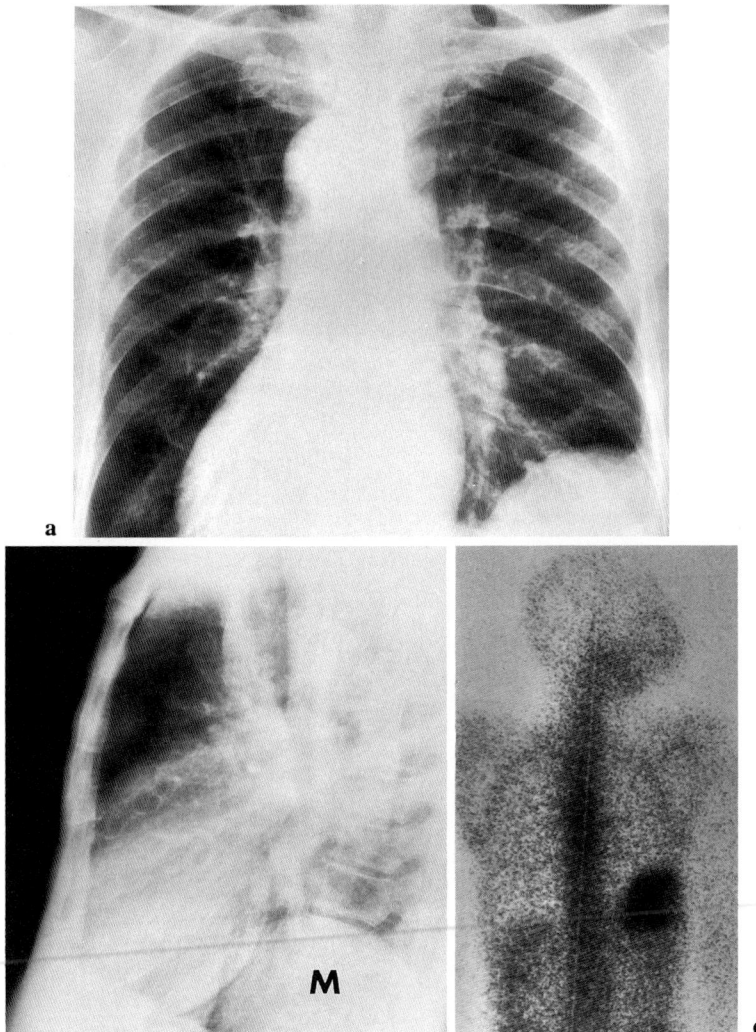

**Fig. 14a–c.** Importance of including a lateral view. **a** Pseudoeventration of the right hemidiaphragm observed in a frontal view radiograph. **b** Lateral view showed a mass (*M*) behind the heart. **c** A gallium scan showed increased uptake at the level of the mass which proved to be a giant cell carcinoma of the lung

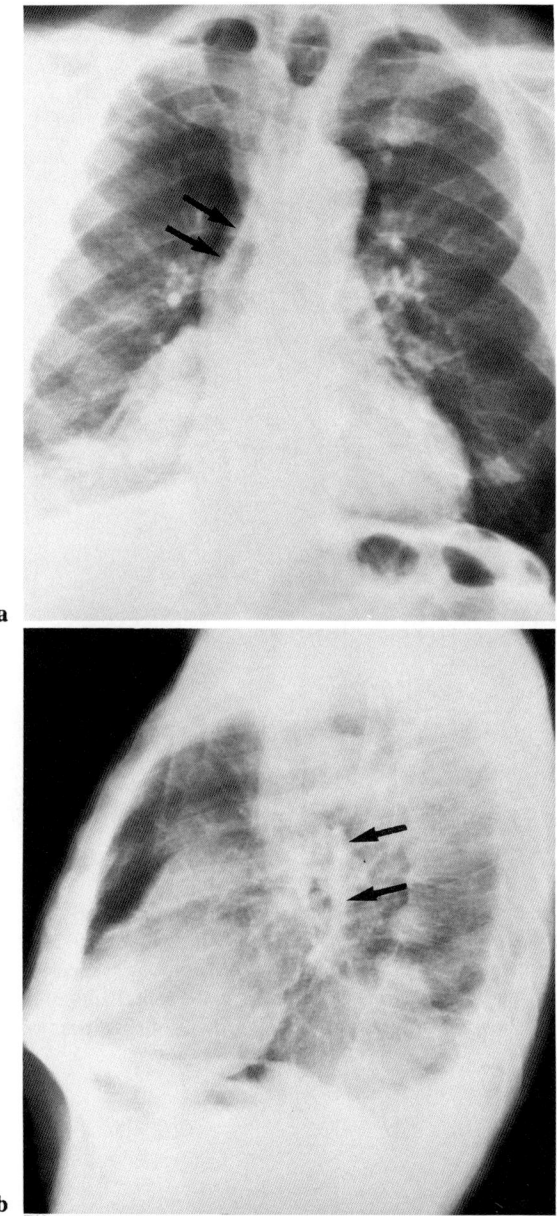

**Fig. 15a, b.** Importance of including a lateral view. **a** Frontal view showed a mass in the right lower lobe. There was thickening of the right tracheal stripe (*arrows*). At endoscopy the mass proved to be a bronchial carcinoma. **b** Lateral view showed thickening of the posterior wall of the bronchus intermedius (*arrows*). This lesion proved to be a nonresectable tumor with invasion of the mediastinum. This finding can be seen in a variety of conditions. However, when observed in a patient with a bronchial carcinoma, should be considered a sign of non-resectability due to mediastinal invasion

32

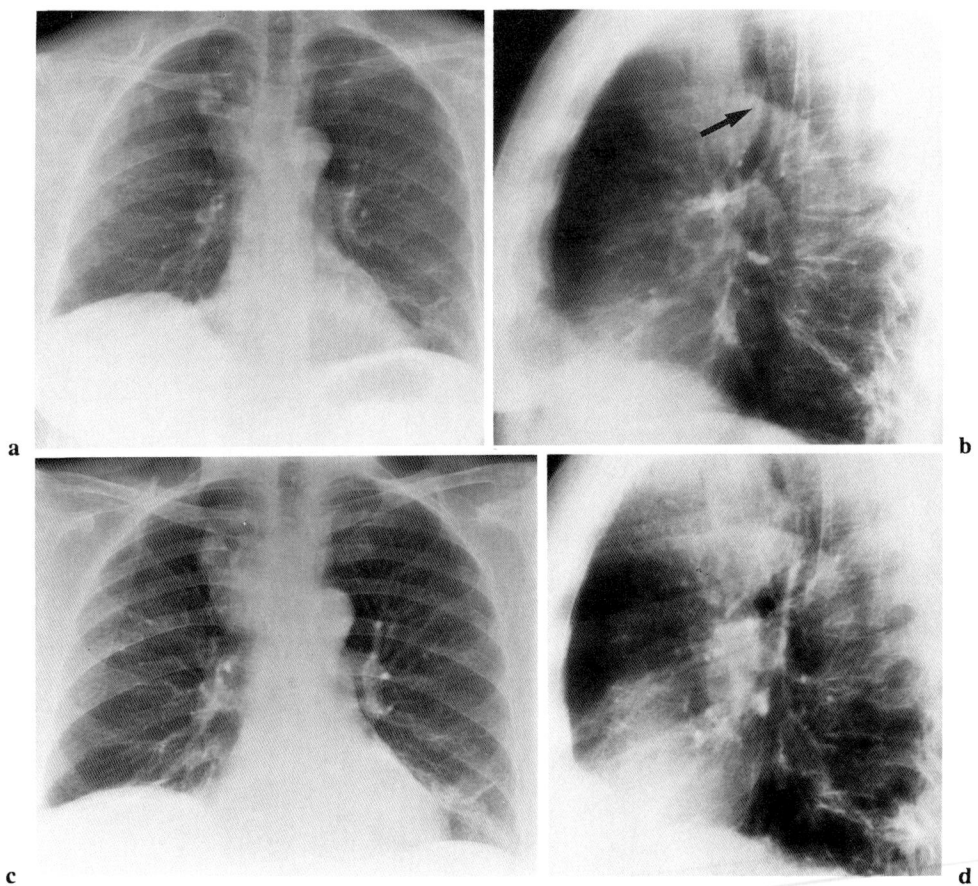

a                                           b

c                                           d

**Fig. 16a–d.** Importance of including a lateral view demonstrated with the example of a tracheal carcinoma. **a** Frontal chest radiograph taken on 26 January 1989. A mass was seen in the right tracheobroncheal angle. A pulmonary process was suspected. **b** The lateral view showed indentation of the anterior trachea (*arrow*). **c, d** Frontal and lateral view radiographs taken on 2 June 1989 showing progression of the growth of this mass which proved to be a tracheal carcinoma

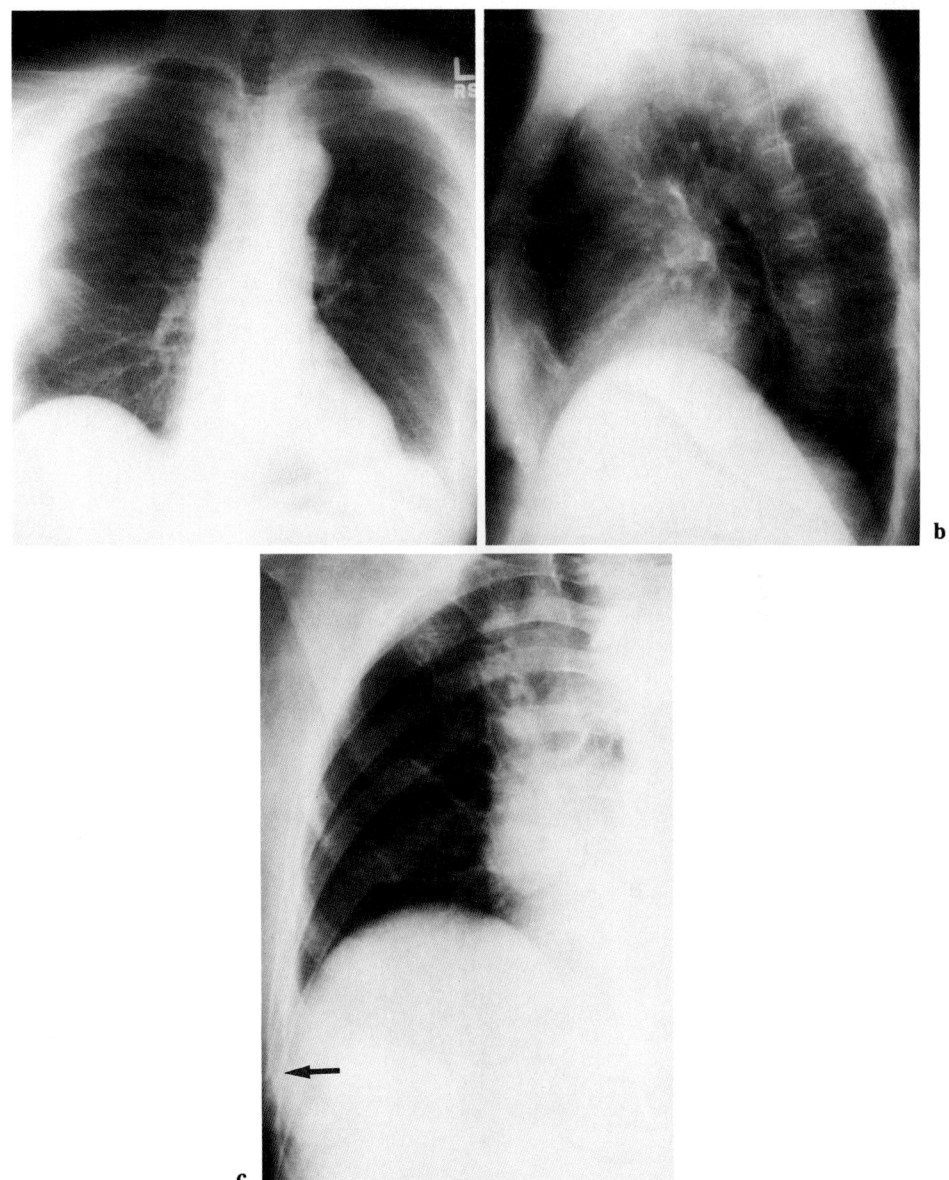

**Fig. 17a–c.** Importance of including an oblique projection. The patient was hit on the right chest. **a** Frontal view of the chest shows an ill-defined density along the right chest wall. **b** A lateral view which was unremarkable. **c** An oblique view showed a rib fracture (*arrow*) not detected on the two previous views

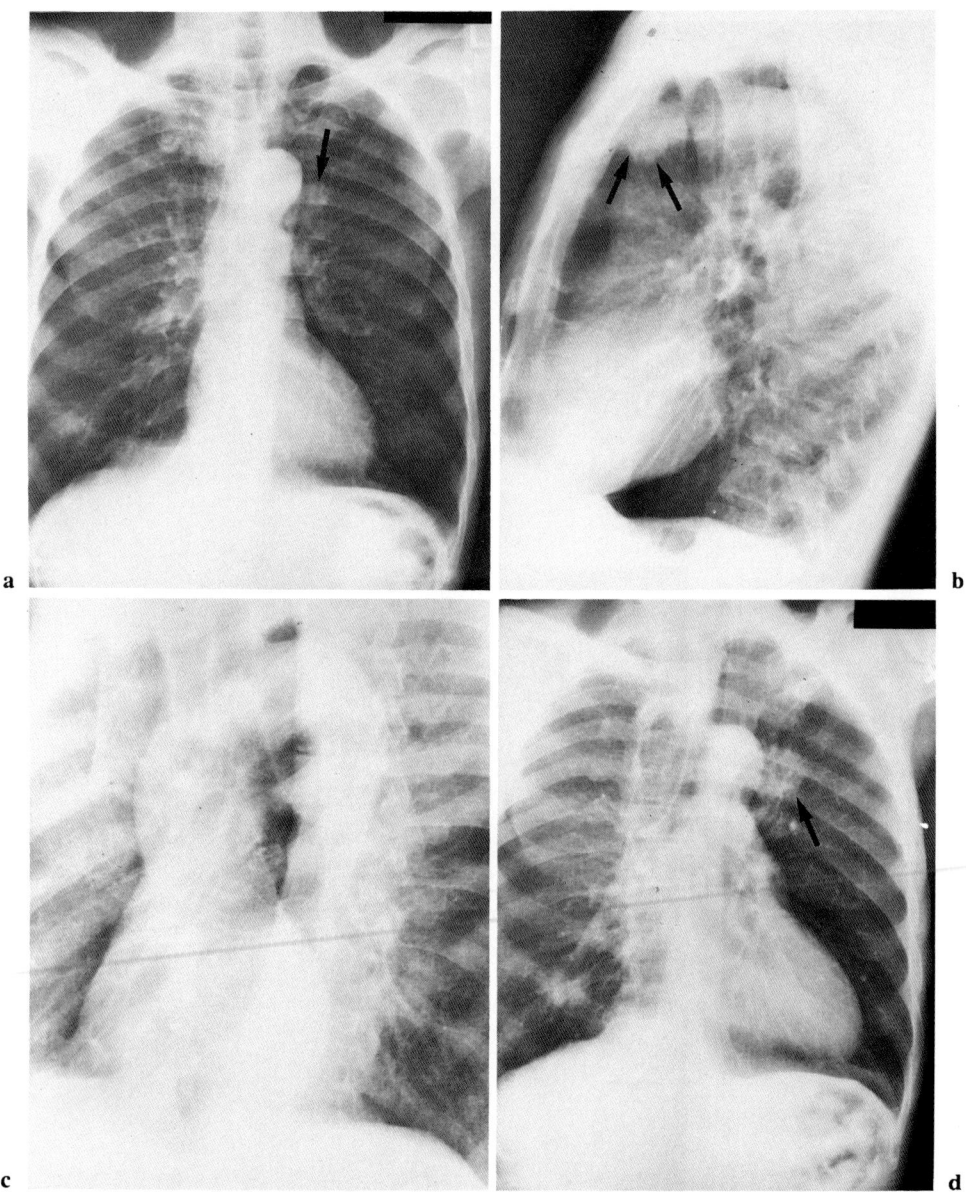

**Fig. 18a–d.** Chest radiographs of a patient with a bronchogenic carcinoma, showing the importance of including oblique views. **a** A frontal view of the chest showing an ill-defined density to the left of the aortic knob (*arrow*). **b** A lateral view showing a density behind the sternum in the anterior mediastinum (*arrows*). **c** A left anterior oblique view which was negative. **d** A right anterior oblique view of the chest where a well-defined mass (*arrow*) proved to represent a bronchogenic carcinoma

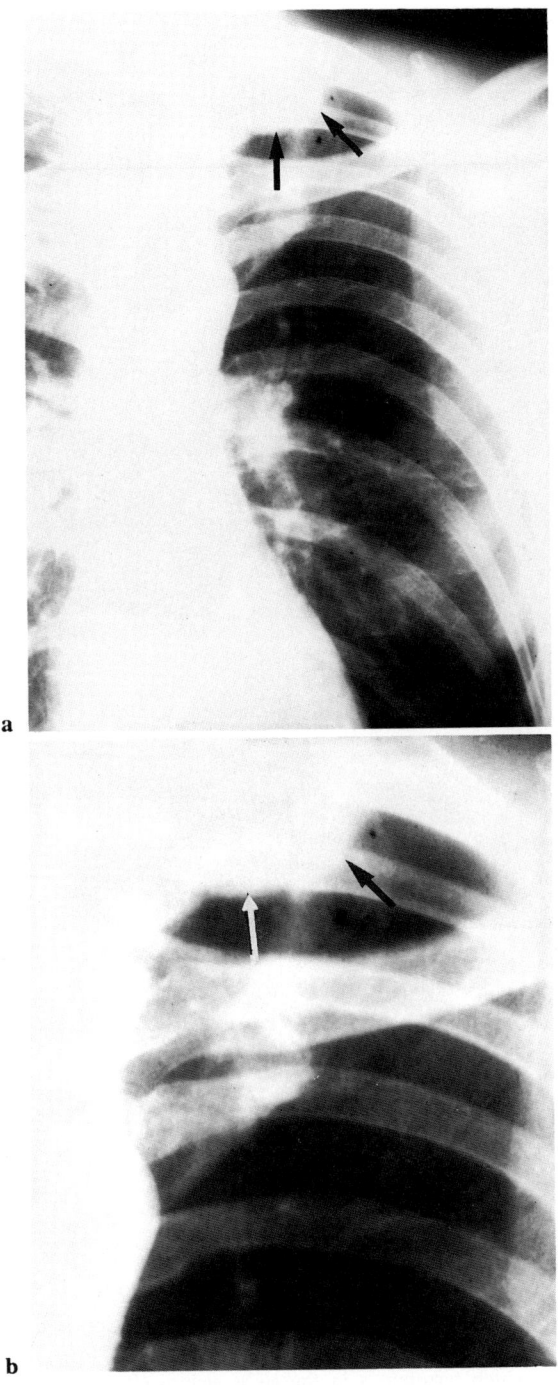

**Fig. 19a, b.** Failure to interpret results correctly. Bronchial carcinoma which was mistaken for focal pleural thickening. **a, b** *Arrows* show the extrapulmonary density in the left apex which proved to represent a bronchial carcinoma

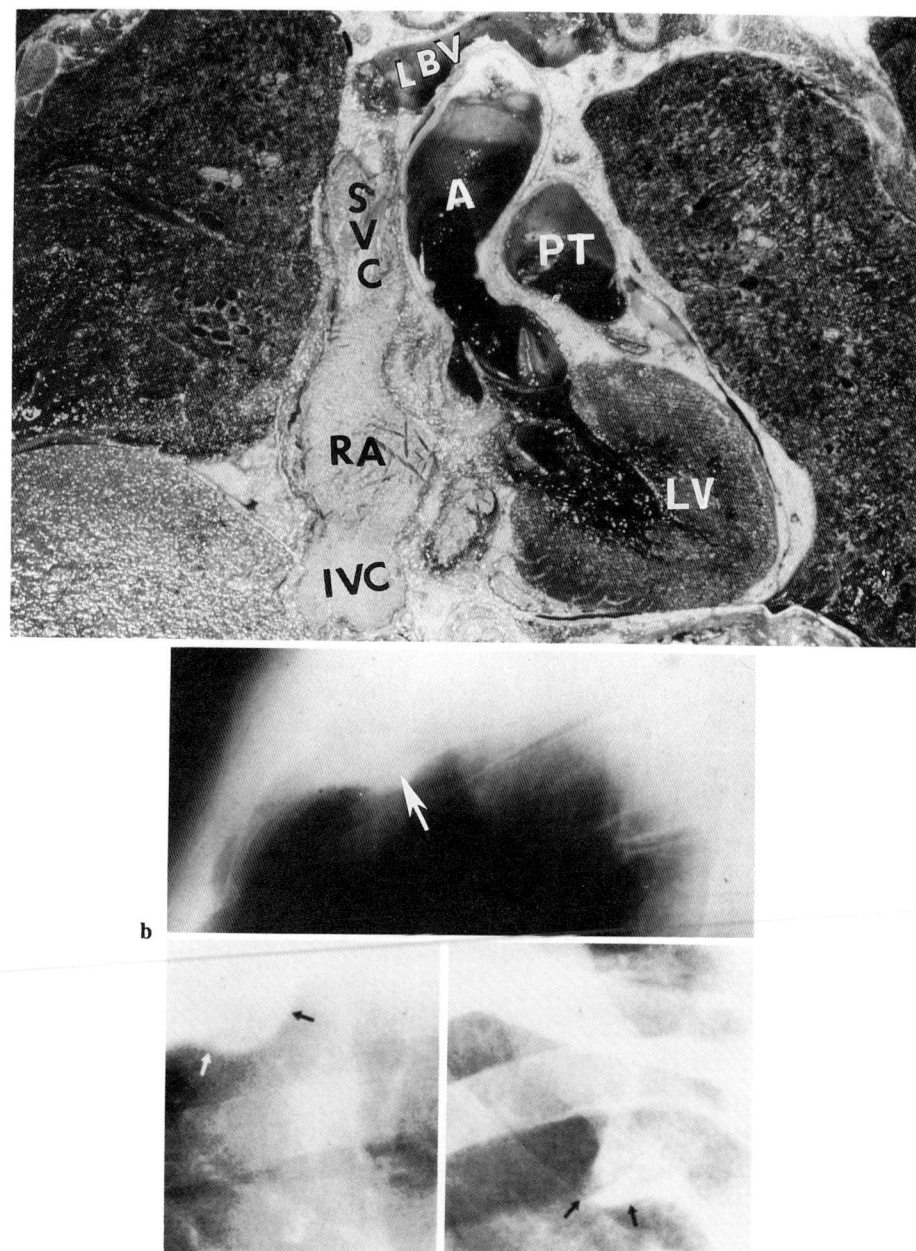

**Fig. 20a–d.** Failure to interpret results correctly. **a** Coronal section at the level of the right atrium. Note left brachiocephalic vein (*LBV*) crossing from left to right to join the superior vena cava (*SVC*) which terminates in the right atrium (*RA*). *IVC*, inferior vena cava; *LV*, left ventricle; *A*, aorta; *PT*, pulmonary trunk. **b** Close-up of the anterior–superior mediastinum. Note extrapulmonary density (*arrow*) which represents the indentation produced by the left brachiocephalic vein. **c, d** The extrapulmonary density in this case corresponded to an osteophyte at the right sternoclavicular joint (*arrows*). Note similarity of findings

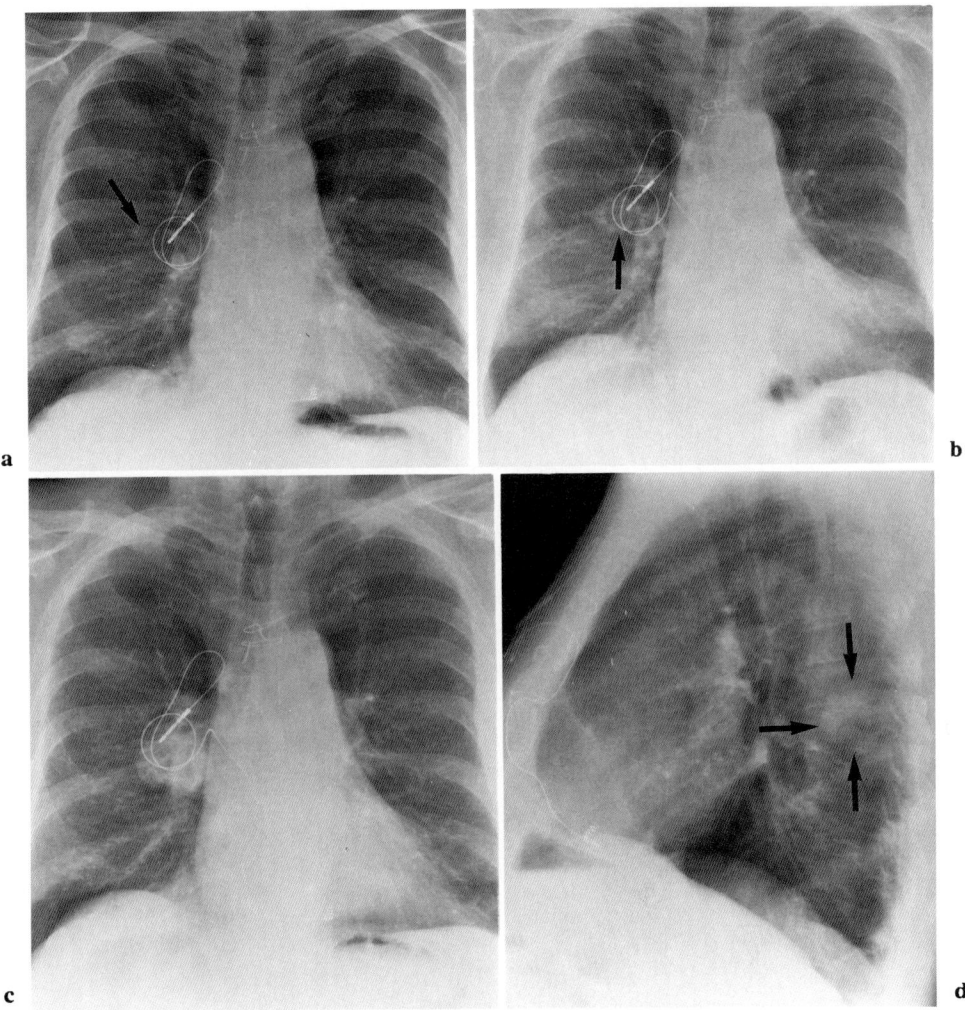

a

b

c

d

**Fig. 21a–d.** Failure to interpret results correctly. Missed bronchial carcinoma. **a** Frontal view radiograph taken on 23 September 1981 revealing a discrete density close to the right hilum (*arrow*). This lesion was overlooked. **b** Frontal view radiograph taken on 23 July 1984, which revealed a small cavity adjacent to the right hilum that was misinterpreted as pneumonia (*arrow*). **c** Frontal view taken on 8 January 1986. **d** Lateral view taken on 22 January 1986. The mass behind the right hilum was best seen in the lateral view radiograph (*arrows*). This lesion proved to be a bronchial carcinoma which had been present since 1981

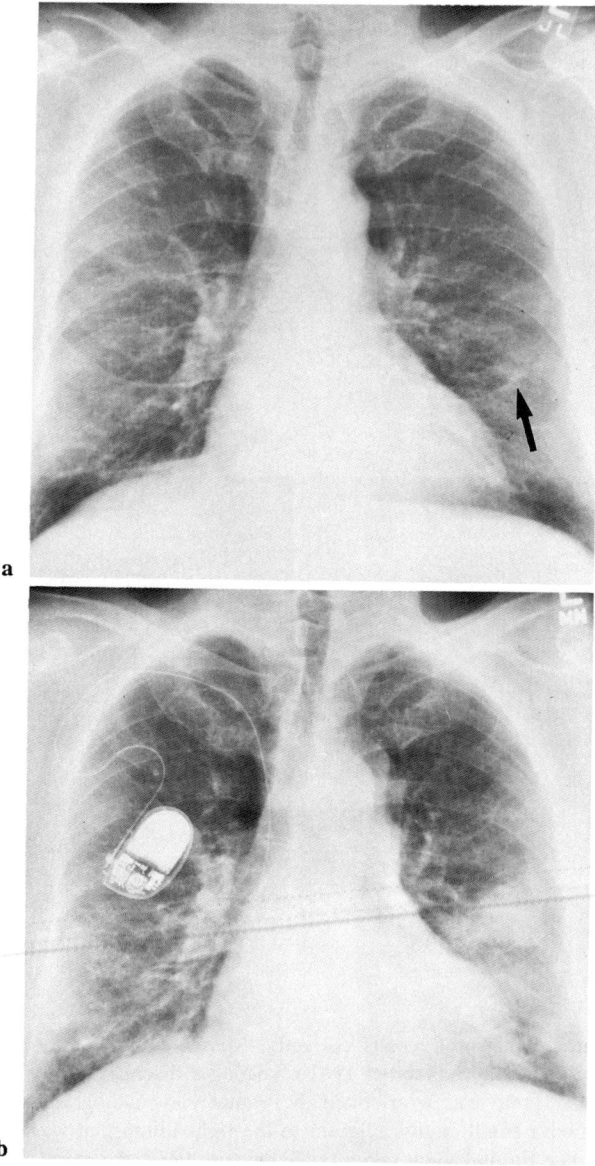

a

b

**Fig. 22a, b.** Failure to interpret results correctly. Missed bronchial carcinoma. **a** A discrete density was observed in the left mid-lung field (*arrow*). This lesion was dismissed by the cardiologist. **b** Film taken 8 months later. Increase in the size of the lesion was noted following the insertion of a pacemaker. The lesion proved to be a bronchial carcinoma, which at this time was nonresectable

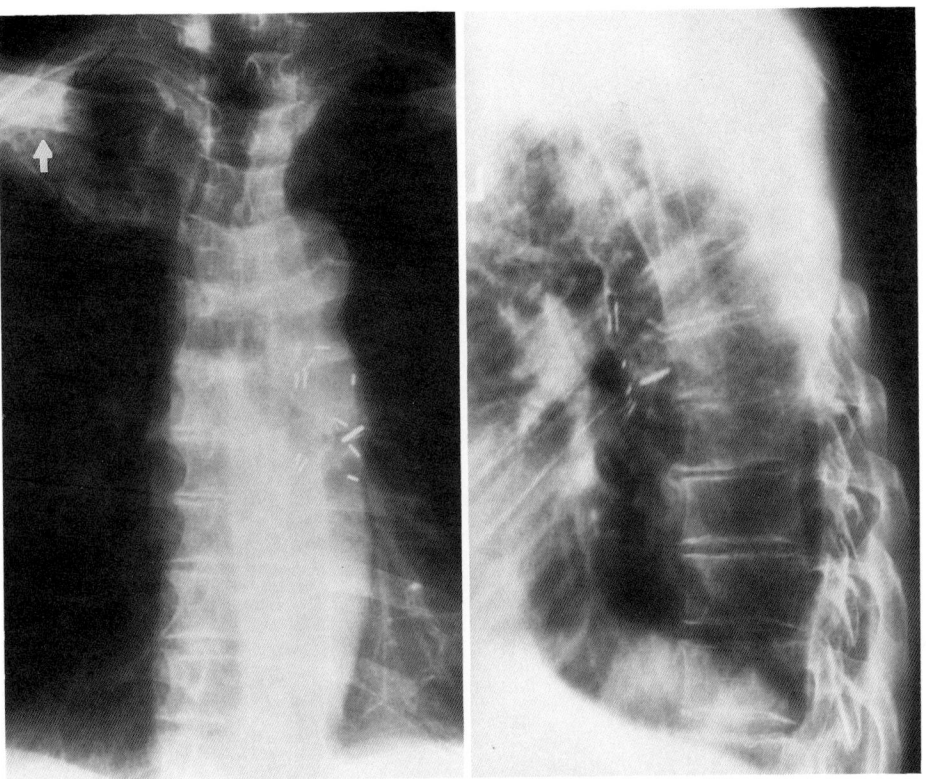

a                                                                                                  b

**Fig. 23a, b.** Failure to interpret results correctly. Missed bronchial carcinoma. **a** Frontal and **b** lateral views revealed a mass at the periphery of the right upper lobe (*arrow*) which was overlooked by the orthopedic surgeon who ordered these two studies and interpreted the films as just showing osteopenia and degenerative changes. There are surgical clips at the level of the left hilum. This lesion represented a bronchial carcinoma

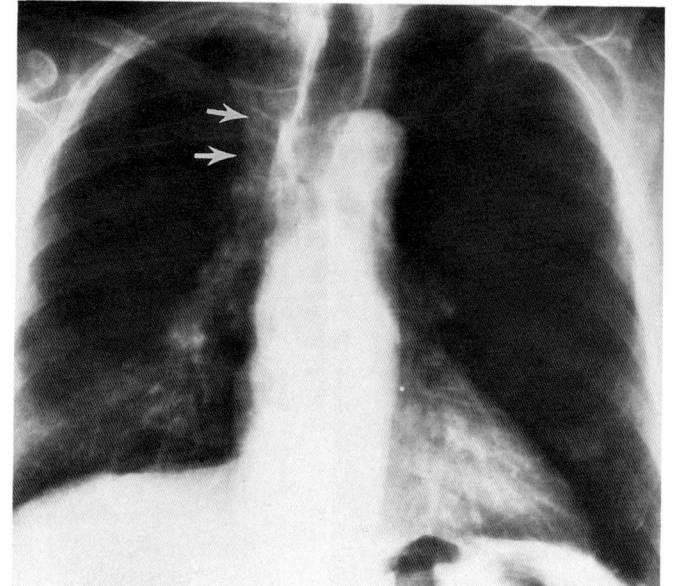

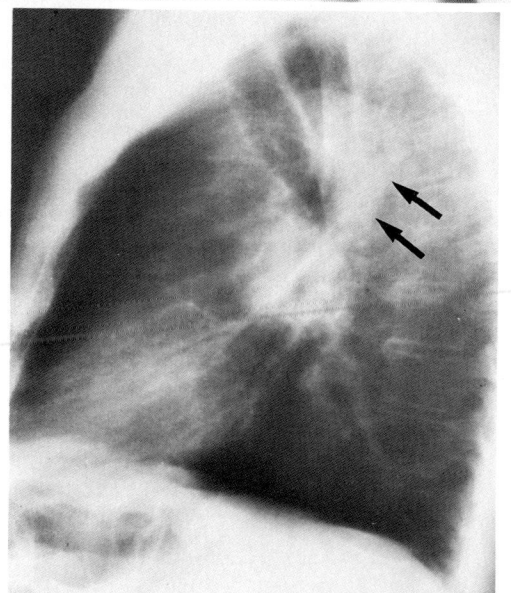

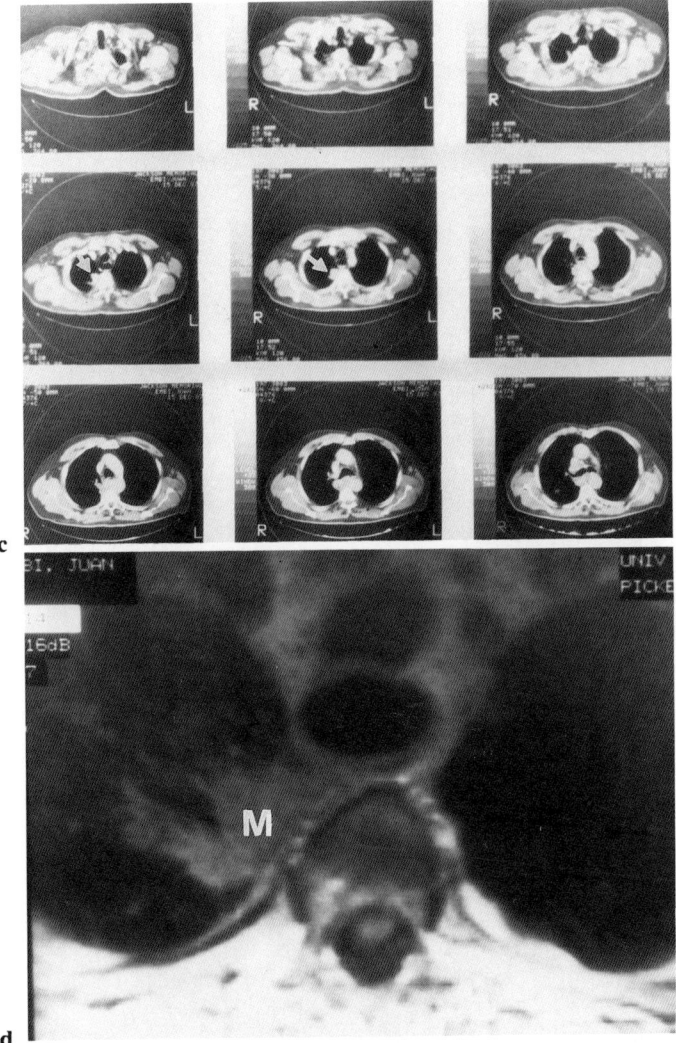

**Fig. 24a–d.** Failure to interpret results correctly. Nonresectable bronchial carcinoma (paravertebral location). **a** Frontal view of the chest. Note an ill-defined density to the right of the trachea (*arrows*). This lesion was overlooked. **b** Lateral view radiograph revealed an ill-defined density below the arch of the aorta (*arrows*). This abnormality was also overlooked. **c** CT examination of the chest revealed a mass in the right paravertebral region (*arrows*). **d** MRI of the upper thoracic region revealing the peripheral mass (*M*) which proved to be a bronchial carcinoma invading the epidural space. This patient presented with back pain and was thought to have osteoarticular disease

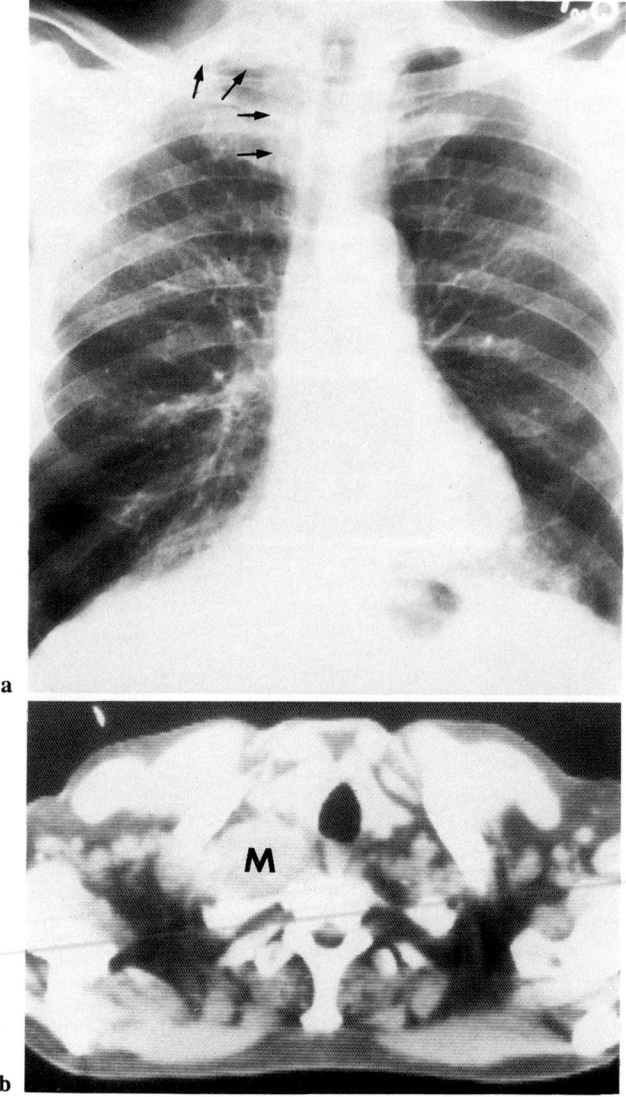

**Fig. 25a, b.** Failure to interpret results correctly. Missed tumor in right paravertebral region (primary neurofibrosarcoma). **a** Frontal view radiograph revealed density to the right of the trachea and also in the right apical region (*arrows*). This was interpreted as fibrosis with pleural thickening. **b** CT revealed a mass (*M*) which proved to be a neurofibrosarcoma

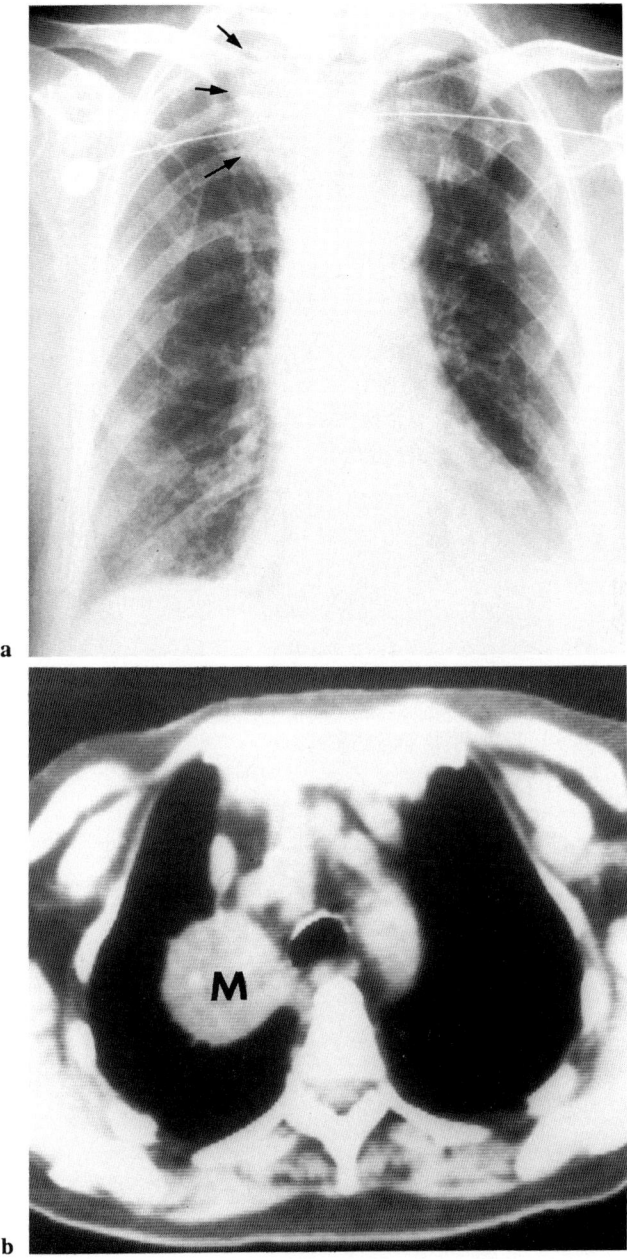

**Fig. 26a, b.** Paraspinal density misinterpreted as tortuous brachiocephalic vessel. **a** Frontal view radiograph showed a slightly enlarged heart and a widened superior mediastinum to the right of the trachea, considered to represent a tortuous brachiocephalic vessel (*arrows*). **b** CT showed a right paratracheal mass (*M*) with calcification. This proved to be metastatic osteosarcoma

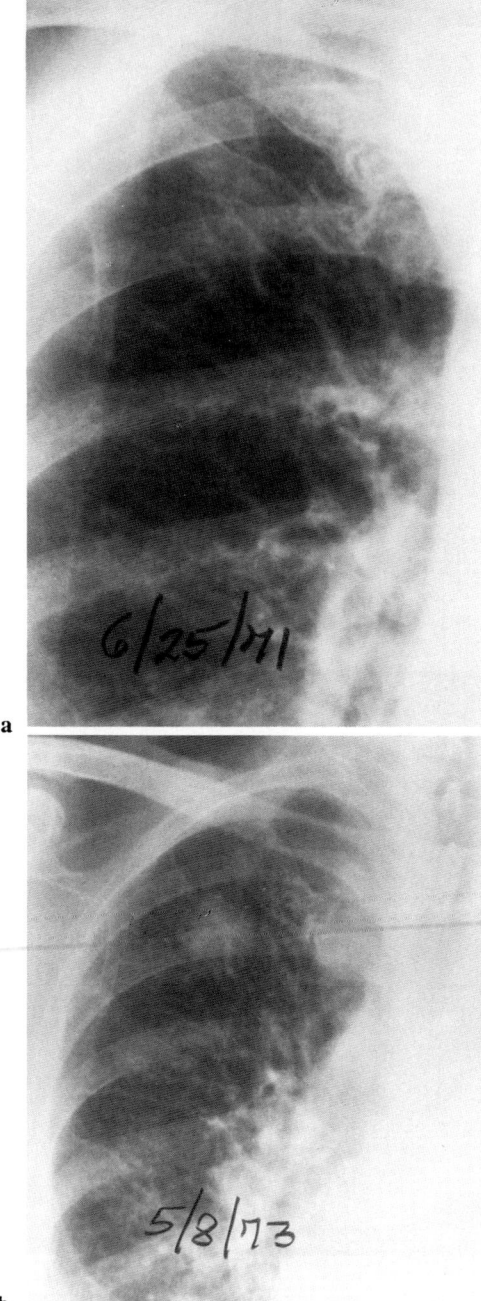

a

b

**Fig. 27a, b.** Failure to diagnose scar carcinoma. **a** Film taken on 25 June 1971 showed linear densities in the right infraclavicular region in a 52-year-old patient who was a heavy smoker. **b** Film taken on 8 May 1973 showing a nodular density which proved to represent a scar carcinoma

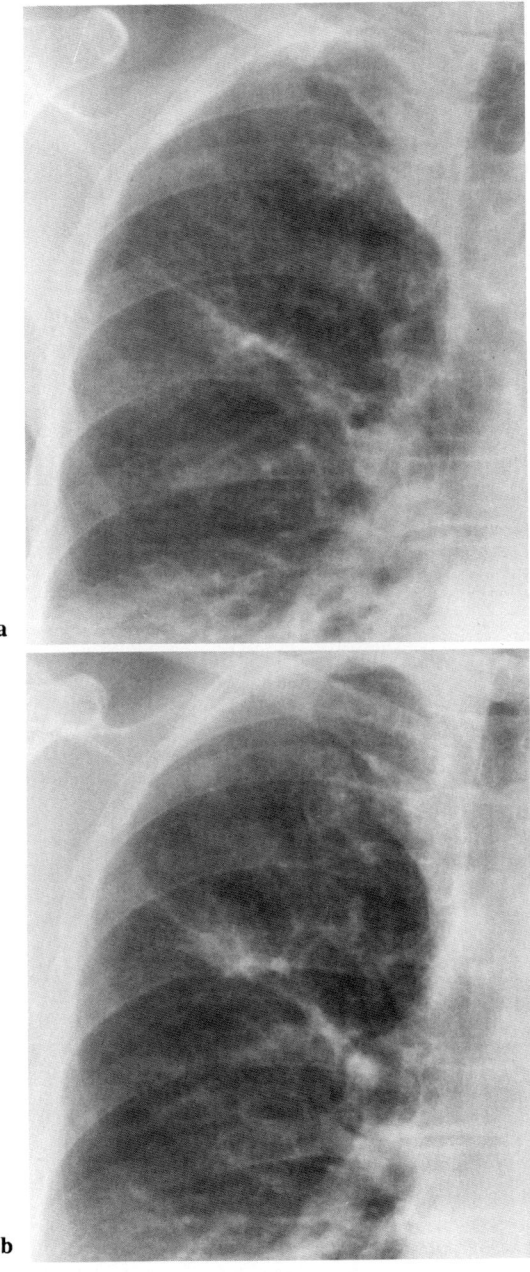

**Fig. 28a, b.** Chest radiographs indicating presence of scar carcinoma. **a** Note scar in upper lobe of the right lung. **b** Note nodular changes at the level of the scar. This irregularity mandated biopsy. The lesion proved to represent bronchioloalveolar cell carcinoma (scar carcinoma). Any changes in the size and/or morphology of a pulmonary scar should be considered a possible scar carcinoma. This and small nodular carcinomas are the pulmonary cancers which are usually cured by surgery

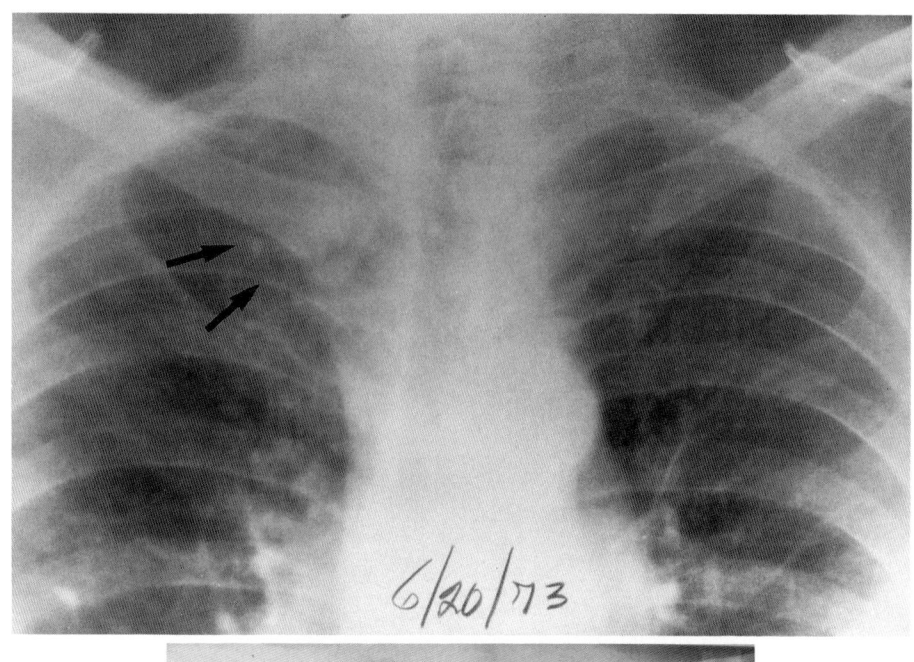

a

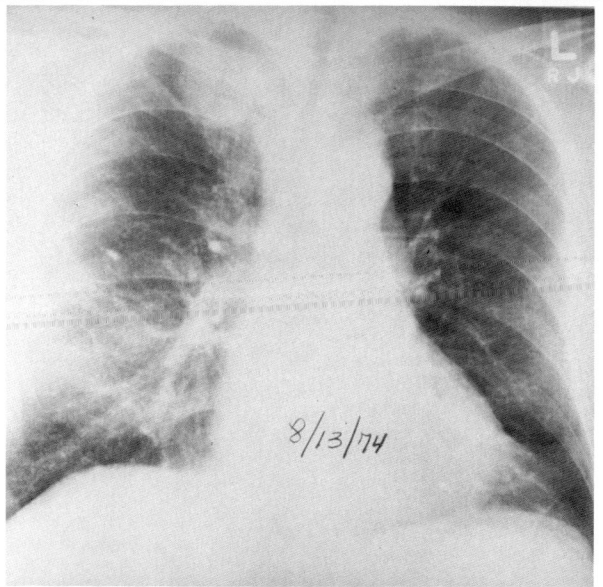

b

**Fig. 29a, b.** Chest radiographs of patient with scar carcinoma. **a** Film taken on 20 June 1973. Note fibrocalcific changes just below the right inner clavicle. **b** Radiograph obtained on 13 August 1974 showing a mass which proved to represent a scar carcinoma

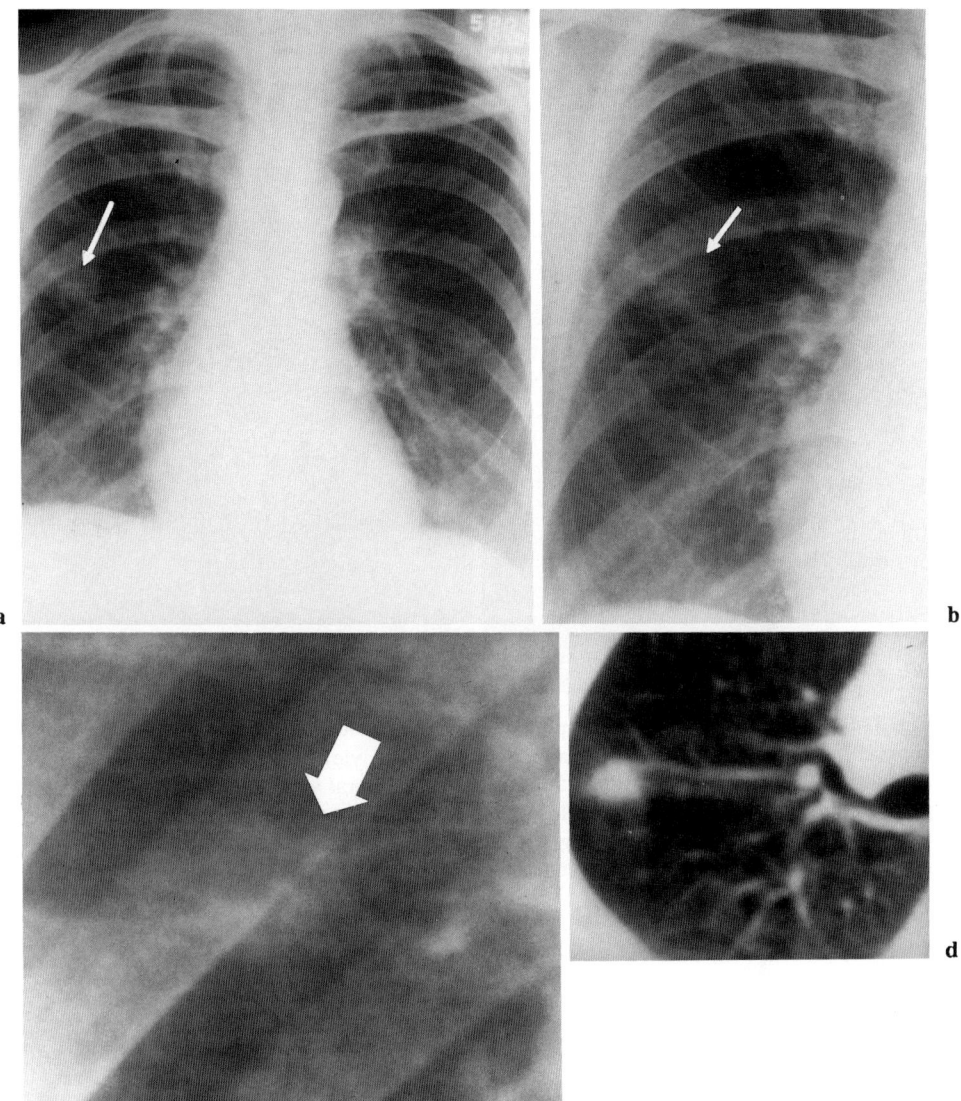

**Fig. 30a–d.** Chest radiographs of patient with scar carcinoma. **a** Frontal view radiograph showing discrete density in right mid-lung field (*arrow*). **b** Close-up of right lung showing linear and nodular changes (*arrow*). **c** Magnification of right lung lesion showing irregular shadow (*arrow*). **d** CT examination showing irregular density connected by linear strands to the right hilum. This lesion proved to be a bronchioloalveolar cell carcinoma associated with a scar

48

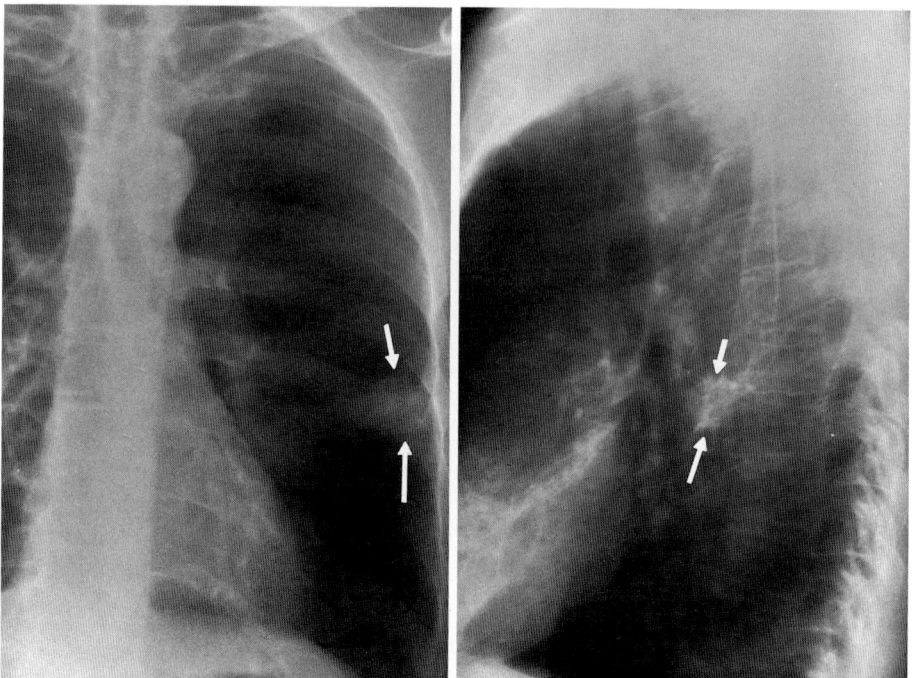

a                                                                                                 b

**Fig. 31a–e.** Calcified lesion misinterpreted as an inflammatory process and which proved to represent a bronchioloalveolar cell carcinoma. **a** Frontal view chest radiograph revealed an irregular density in the left mid-lung field (*arrows*). **b** Lateral view. **c** Close-up of the frontal projection of the lesion (*arrows*). **d** Close-up of a lateral view of the chest showing the lesion (*arrows*). **e** CT examination showing irregular shadow with focal pleural thickening. This proved to be a bronchioloalveolar cell carcinoma arising in an area of scarring. Irregular califications were present

Some general statistical information on the incidence of scar carcinoma of the lung (from Bakris 1983):

– Found in 1% of autopsied patients and 7% of lung tumors.
– 45% of all peripheral cancers originated in a scar.
– 72% of all scar carcinomas were adenocarcinomas and 18% were squamous cell carcinomas. The rest were undifferentiated large cell carcinomas. None was of oat cell or small cell type.
– Over 75% of all scar carcinomas were found in the upper lobes.
– More than 50% or all scar carcinomas were related to infarcts.
– Less than 25% were related to tuberculosis scars.

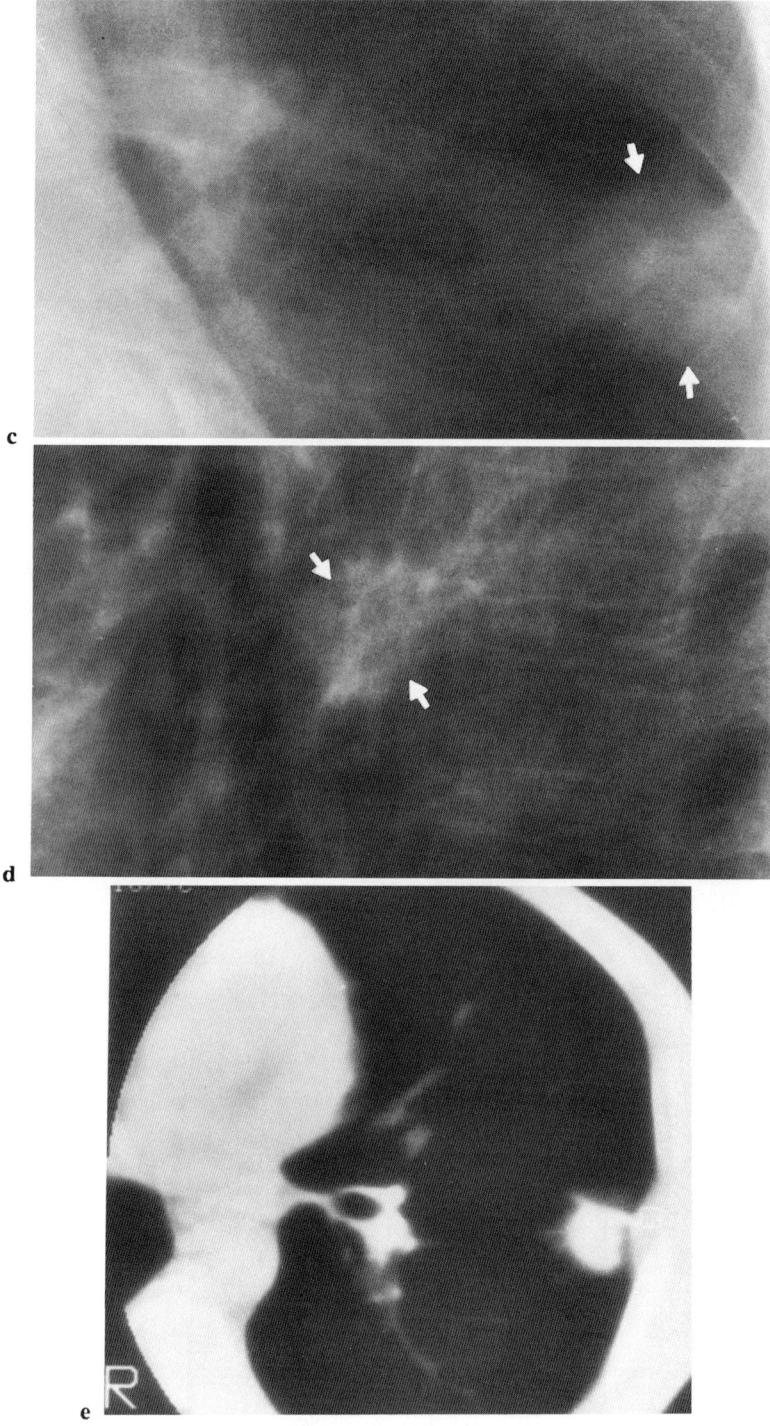

c

d

e

50

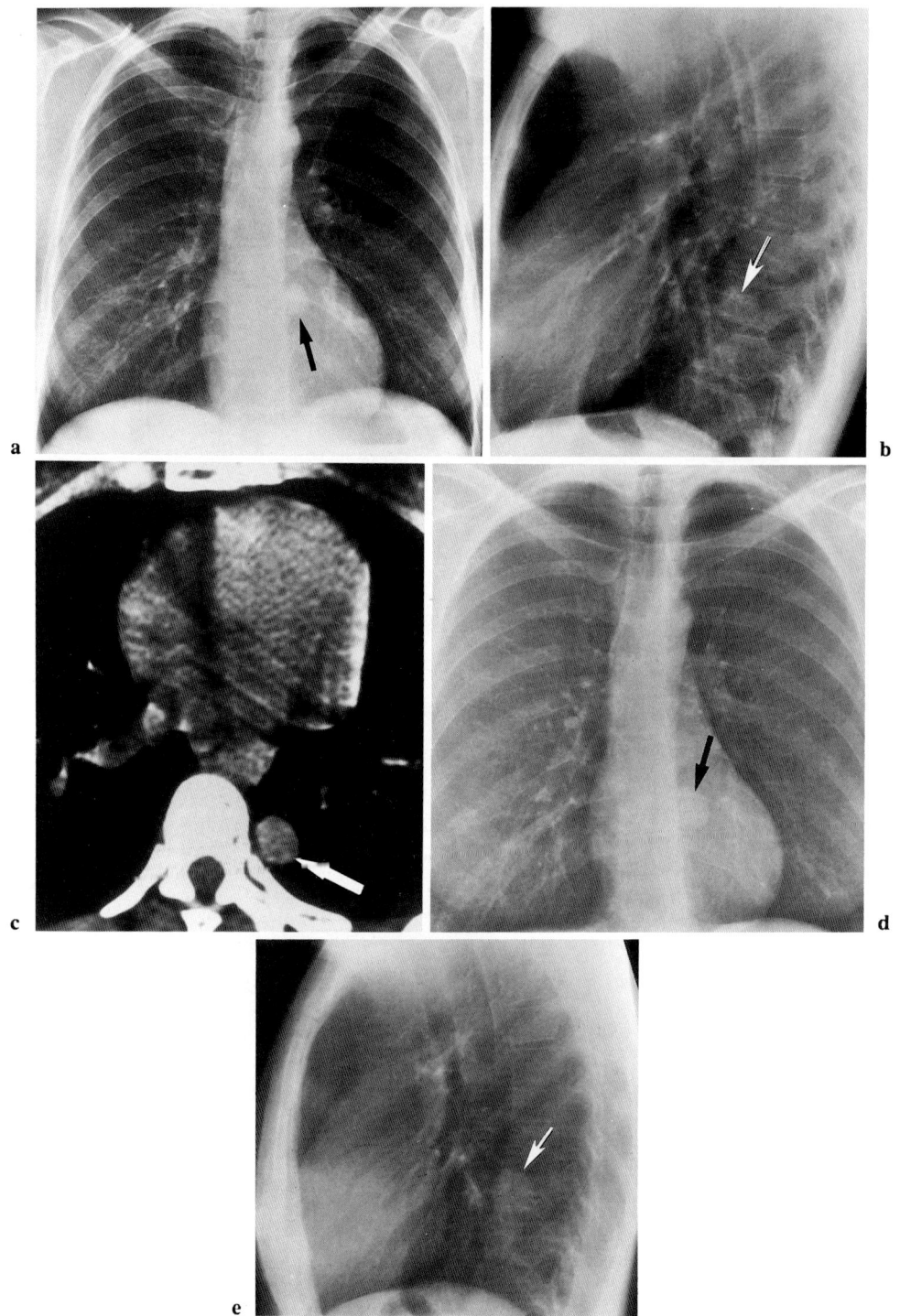

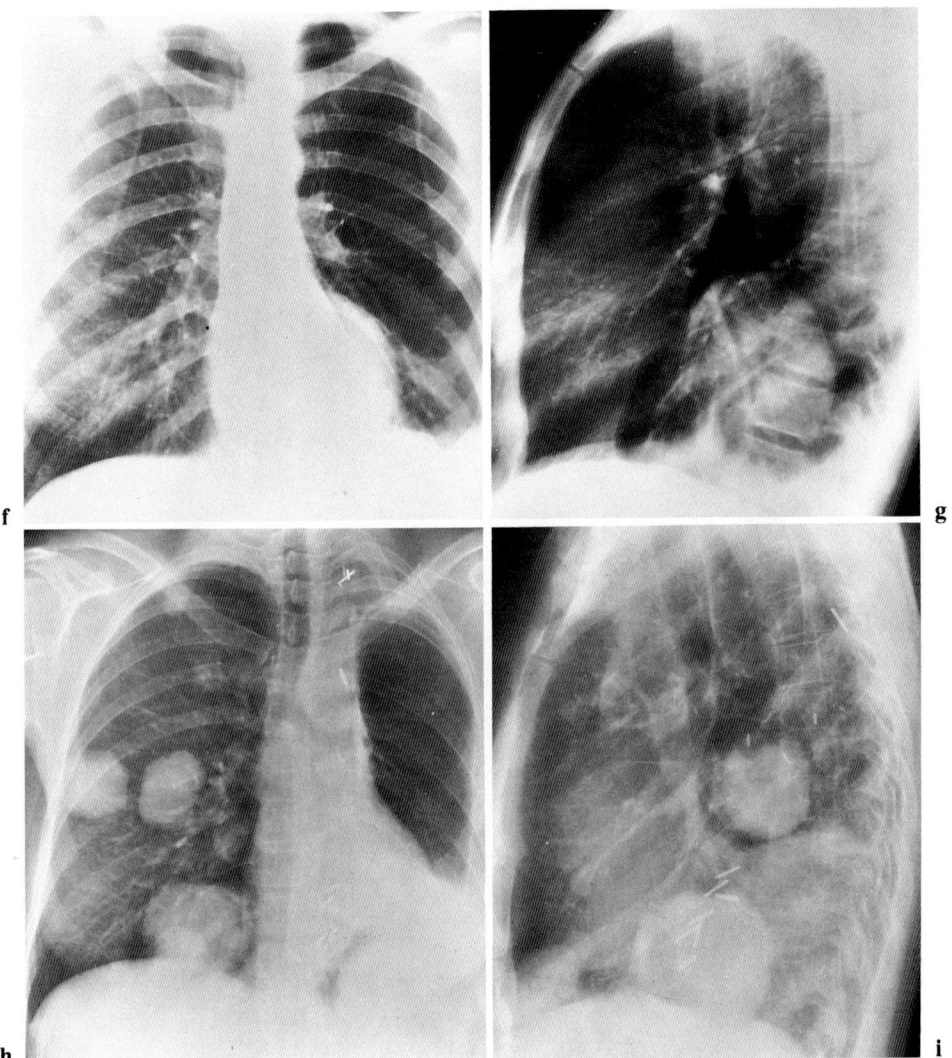

Fig. 32a–i. Primary hemanigopericytoma which was thought to be a granuloma. a Frontal view chest radiograph taken on 10 September 1984 revealing nodule behind the heart (*arrow*). b Lateral view radiograph showing nodule superimposed on a thoracic vertebral body (*arrow*). c CT examination showing nodule with scattered calcific deposits (*arrow*). d Frontal view chest radiograph taken on 18 December 1984 showing unchanged pulmonary nodule (*arrow*). e Lateral view chest radiograph showing nodule ajacent to vertebral body (*arrow*). Because the lesion was calcified it was thought to represent a benign process in this 28-year-old asymptomatic woman. The woman did not follow instructions to return for tissue diagnosis and close follow-up. A frontal view chest radiograph (f) and a lateral view chest radiograph (g) were taken a year and a half later. Note considerable enlargement of the mass. Frontal (h) and lateral (i) view chest radiographs showing post-thoracotomy changes and multiple "cannonball" metastasis. The lesion proved to probably be a primary hemangiopericytoma. It was called primary synovial sarcoma by the Armed Forces Institute of Pathology, Washington, D.C. When calcifications in a mass are irregularly dispersed, the lesion can be either benign or malignant. Only when the mass is uniformly calcified it is to be considered a benign lesion

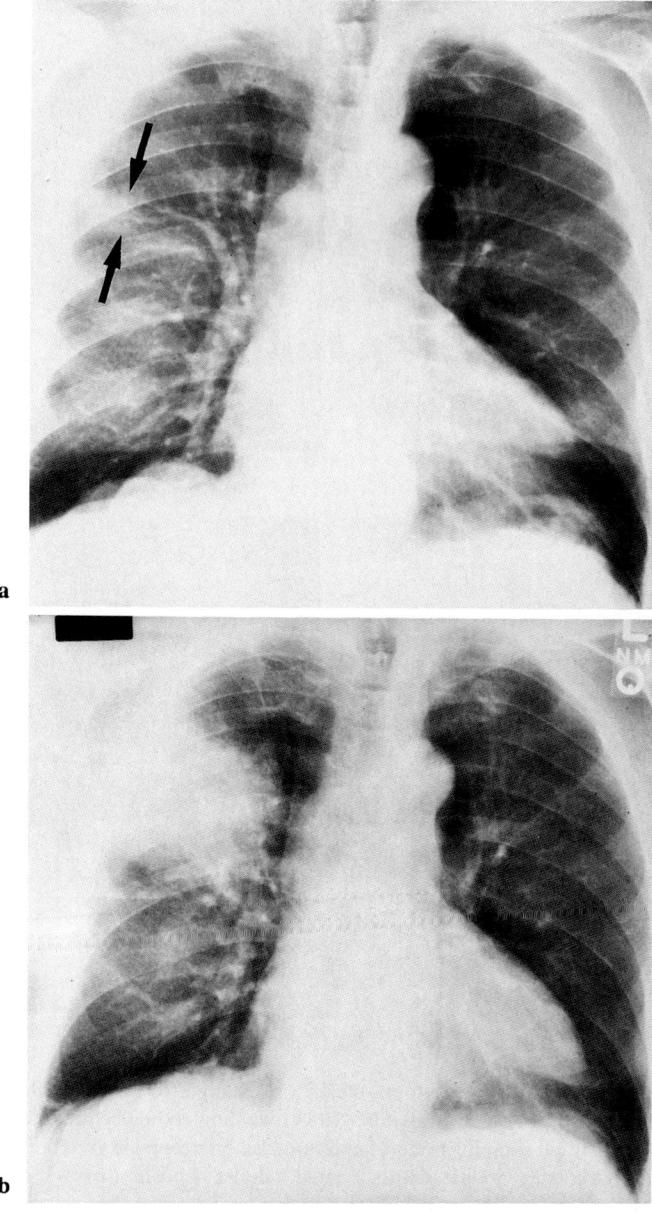

a

b

**Fig. 33a, b.** Small bronchial carcinoma which was mistaken for anterior end of a rib. **a** Frontal view chest radiograph of an 82-year-old man with cardiomegaly. A discrete density in the periphery of the upper lobe of the right lung was mistaken for the anterior end of a rib (*arrows*). **b** Follow-up chest radiograph taken a year and a half later. Note explosive growth of a bronchial carcinoma. The lesion was larger than the rib, therefore it should have been recognized as a lesion. The cardiologist of this patient ignored the recommendation of the radiologist for further studies when the lesion was initially suspected

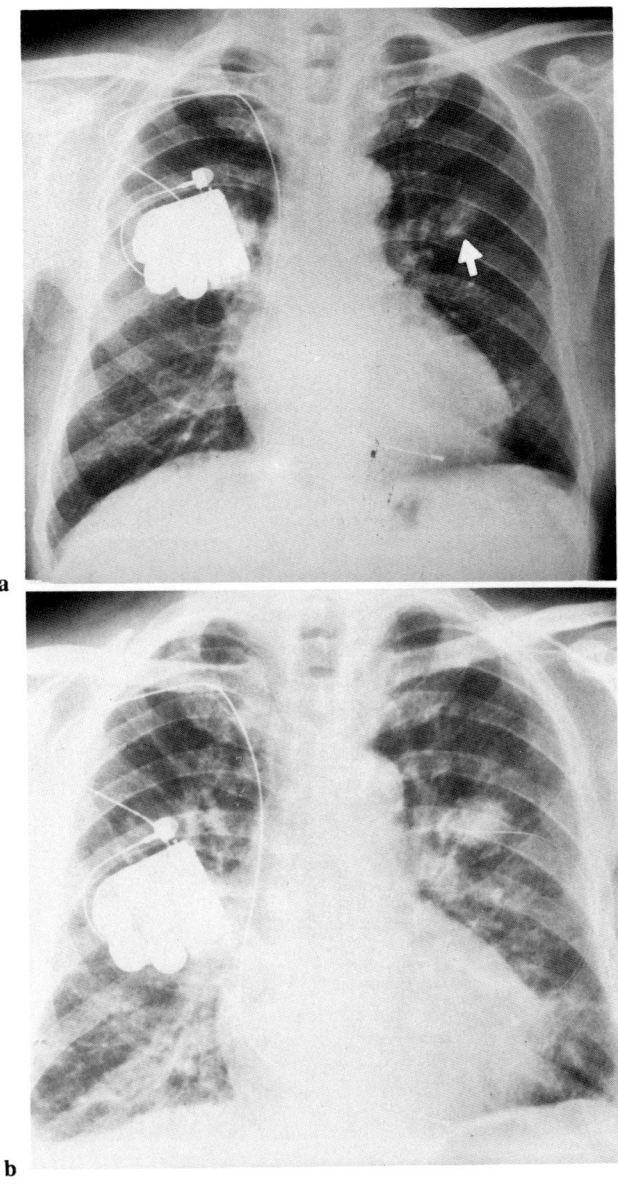

a

b

**Fig. 34a, b.** Bronchial carcinoma missed in a patient with cardiac disease. **a** Elderly gentle-man with cardiac arrythmia. At the time of pacemaker insertion, a chest radiograph revealed a discrete density in the mid-portion of the left lung (*arrow*). This lesion was overlooked. **b** Frontal view chest radiograph taken a year later. Note growth of the bronchial carcinoma

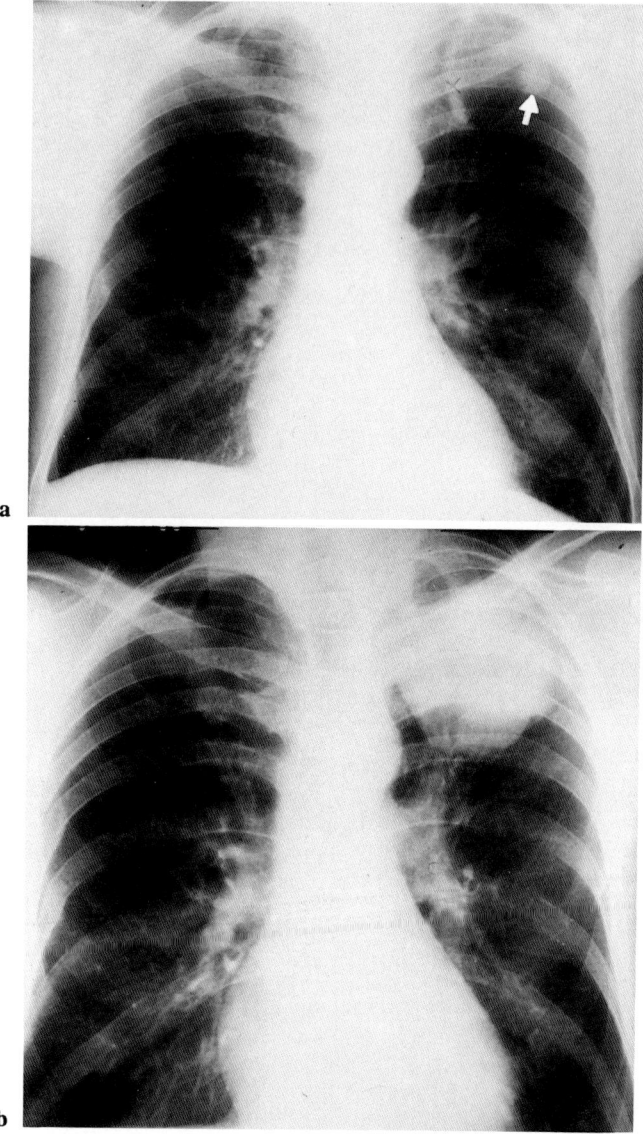

a

b

**Fig. 35a, b.** Solitary mulmonary nodule which was overlooked. **a** Frontal view chest radiograph taken at an internist's office. A nodule in the left infraclavicular region was missed (*arrow*). There was a scar in the medial aspect of the left upper lobe (*X*). **b** Film taken 3 years later. Note a large bronchial carcinoma which had spread to the left hilum

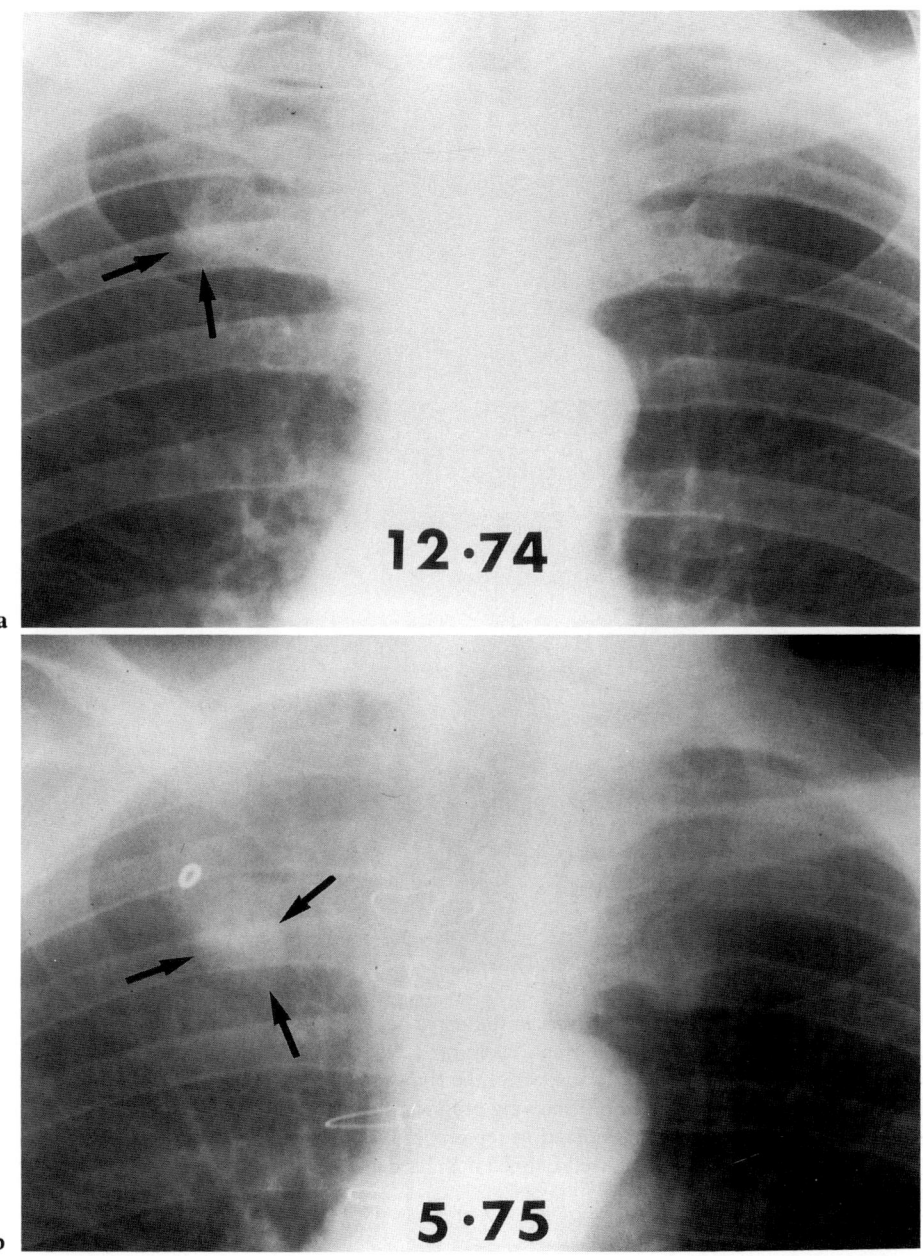

**Fig. 36a, b.** Small bronchial carcinoma mistaken for an osteophyte. **a** Film taken in December 1974 shows a discrete density projecting below the anterior aspect of the right first rib (*arrows*). This was interpreted as an osteophyte. **b** In May 1975, the lesion became more apparent (*arrows*). Note a marker in the anterior aspect of the right first rib. This proved to be a bronchial carcinoma. (Photographs courtesy of Dr. Paul Friedman, University of California, San Diego, USA). In the film of December 1974 one can see the inferior cortex of the rib. Therefore, the density could not arise from the bone

56

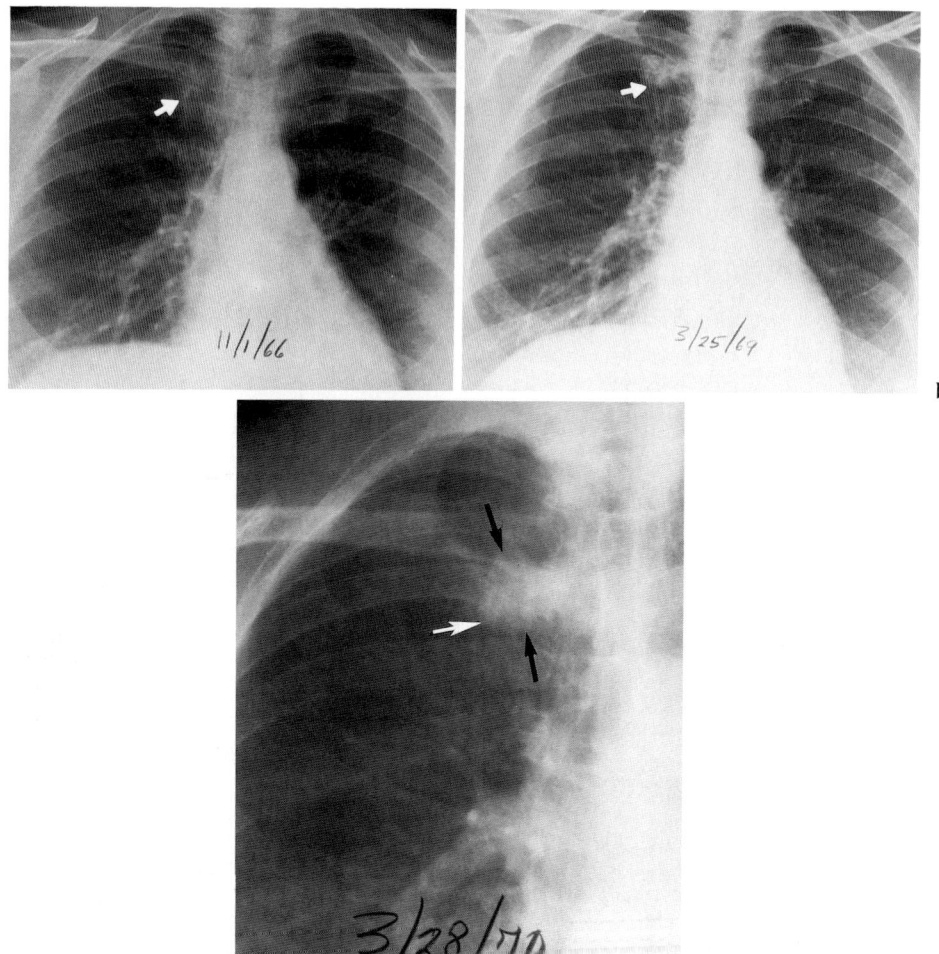

Fig. 37a–c. Small bronchial carcinoma in the upper lobe of the right lung which was over-looked. a Frontal view chest radiograph taken on 1 November 1966. Discrete density was noted superimposed on the anterior aspect of the right first rib (*arrow*). b Frontal view chest radiograph taken on 25 March 1969 showing progressive enlargement of this nodular density (*arrow*). At this time it was considered to represent an osteophyte. c On 28 March 1970, a close-up of this region showed a well-defined nodular density which proved to be a bronchial carcinoma (*arrows*)

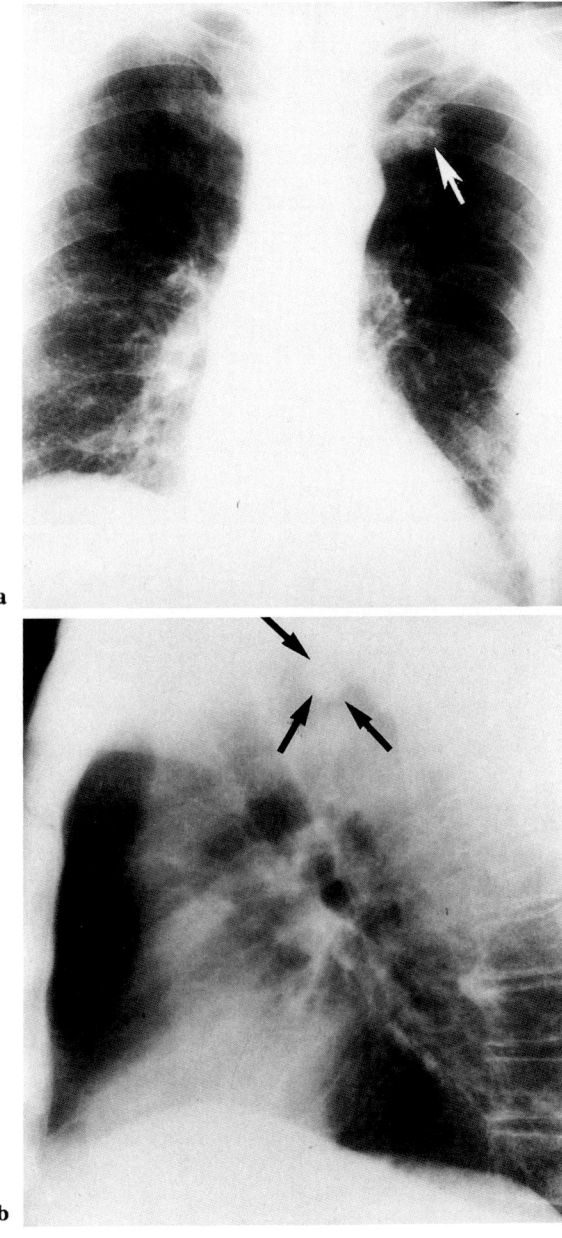

a

b

**Fig. 38a, b.** Nodule in the upper lobe of the left lung missed by internist. **a** Frontal view chest radiograph showing discrete nodular density projecting at the level of the anterior arch of the left first rib (*arrow*). This study was reported as negative. **b** Lateral view chest radiograph showing nodule above the aortic arch. It proved to be a bronchial carcinoma (*arrows*)

58

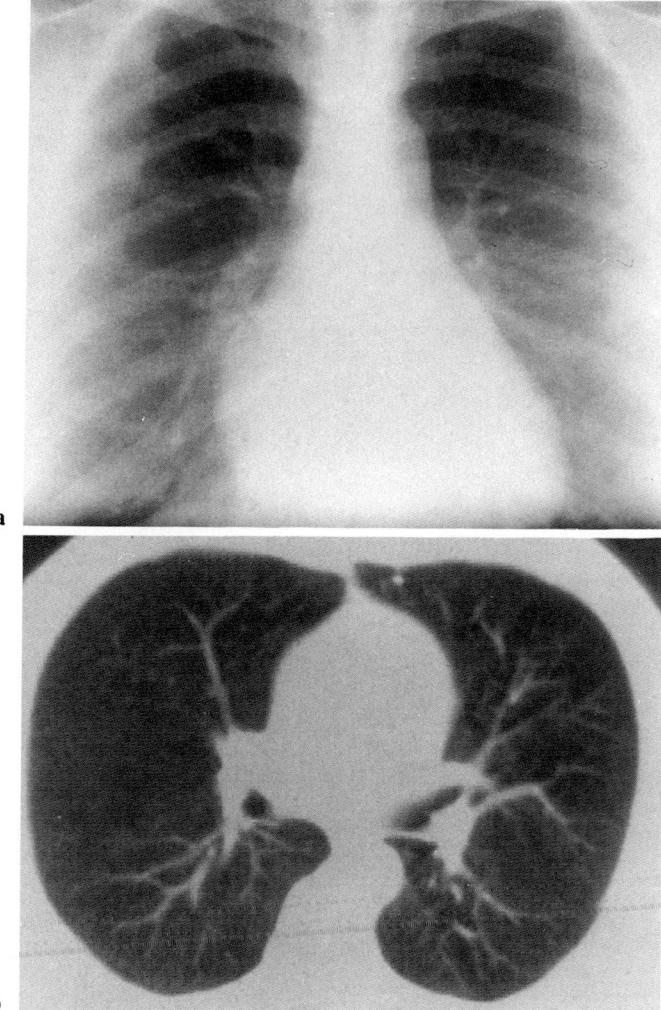

**Fig. 39a, b.** Normal hyperlucency in mid-portion of the right lung which is often misinterpreted. **a** Frontal view chest radiograph showing right mid-lung radiolucency. **b** CT image showing paucity of vascularity in right mid-lung field. This is a normal anatomical finding which should not be interpreted as emphysema or pulmonary embolism

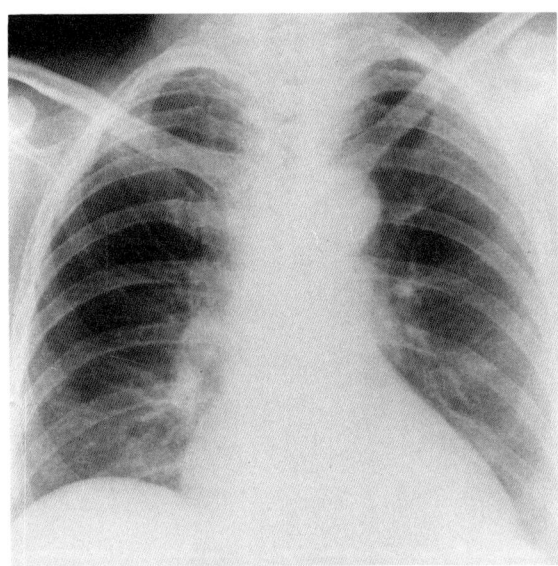

**Fig. 40.** Hyperlucency which is often misinterpreted. Postmastectomy changes. Right mid-lung field appeared hyperlucent. The patient's right breast had been removed. Simple and radical mastectomies can account for unilateral hyperlucencies

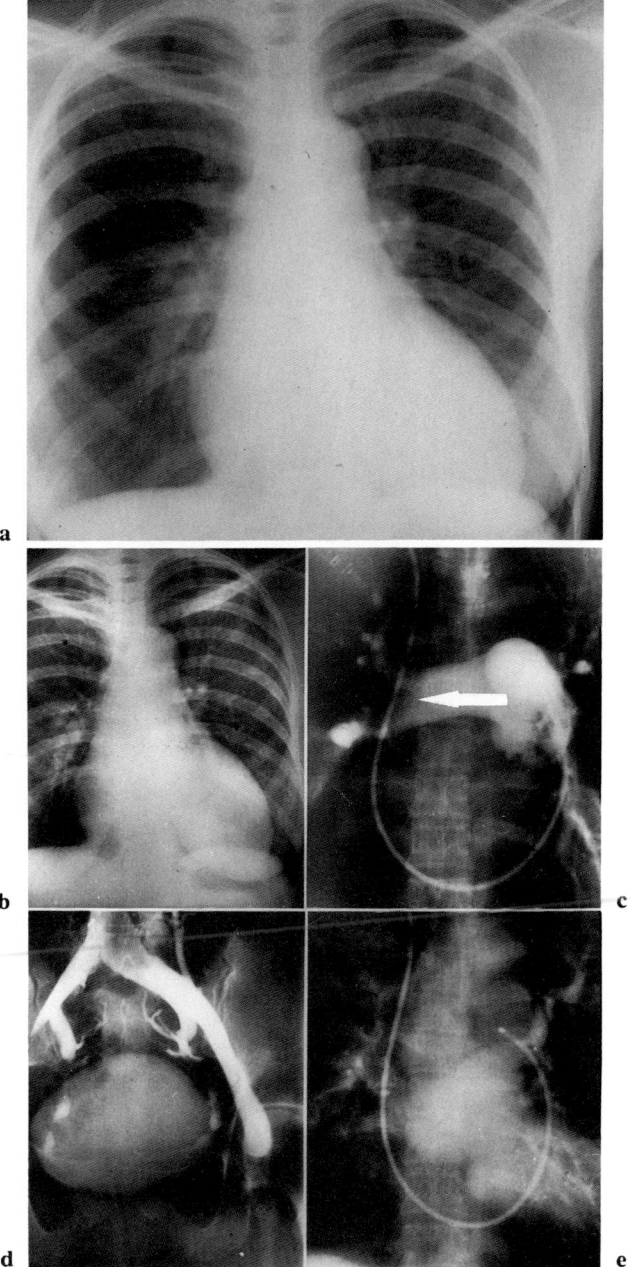

a

b                                    c

d                                    e

**Fig. 41a–e.** Hyperlucency which is often not recognized or misinterpreted. Right mid-lung field lucency due to pulmonary embolism. **a** Frontal view radiograph showed enlargement of the heart, prominent right pulmonary artery, and localized hyperlucency in right mid-lung field. **b, c** Close-up showed that the hyperlucency was related to a saddle thrombus at the bifurcation of the right pulmonary artery (*arrow*). **d** A radiograph of the inferior vena cava showed irregularities in the iliac veins which were the site of the emboli. **e** Late phase of pulmonary angiogram. In a patient with unexplained tachypnea, chest pain and/or low arterial oxygen saturation, localized hyperlucency should be interpreted as possible pulmonary embolism. A perfusion lung scan and angiography should be considered and done promptly

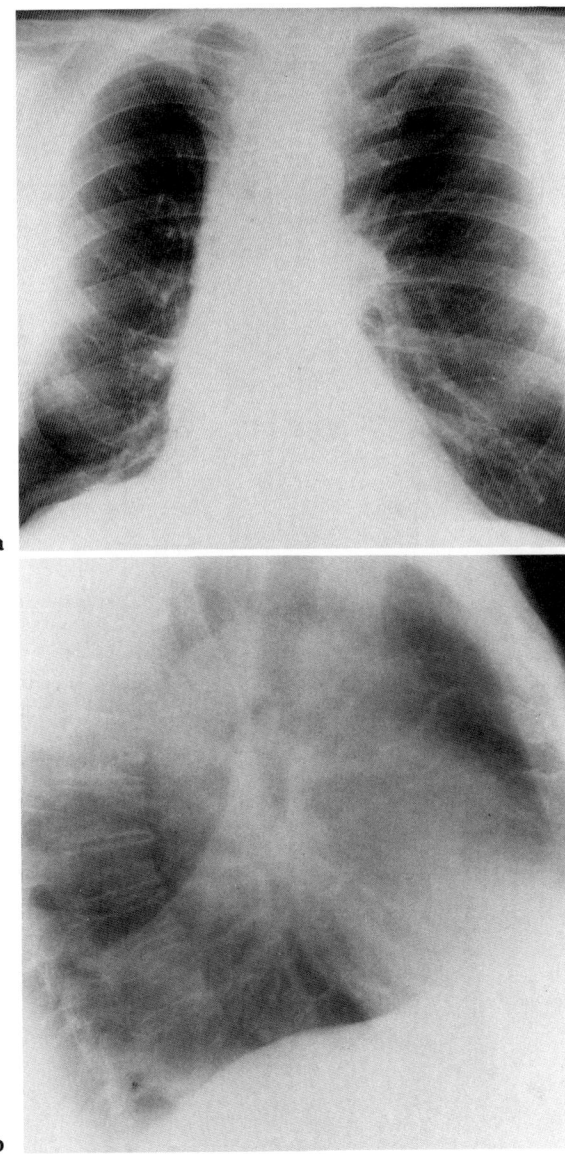

a

b

**Fig. 42a, b.** Hyperlucency as an expression of lobar collapse. Hyperlucency of the right lung was due to collapse of the right lower lobe (**a**). Note the disappearance of the right hilar shadow, the shift of the mediastinum to the right, and the volume loss of the entire right lung. **b** The collapsed right lower lobe is well demonstrated. The hyperlucency is secondary to loss of vascular markings and to the compensatory hyperexpansion of the adjacent lobes

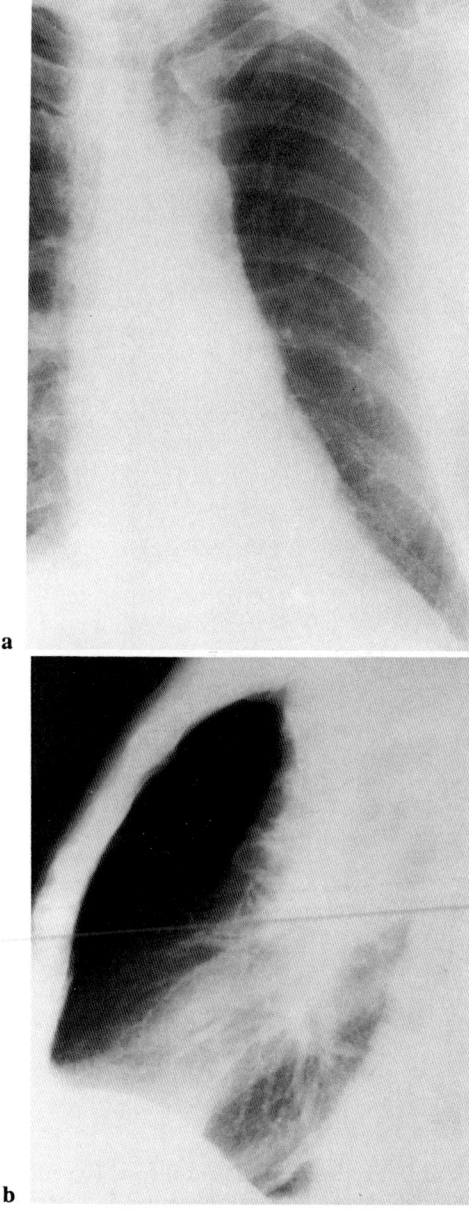

a

b

**Fig. 43a, b.** Hyperlucency due to collapse of the left lower lobe. Hyperlucency of the left lung (a) corresponded to a collapse of the left lower lobe (b). Note in the lateral view that we only see the right hemidiaphragm. There is compensatory hyperexpansion of the left upper lobe. In the frontal view we see loss of the left hilar shadow and paucity of the vascular markings

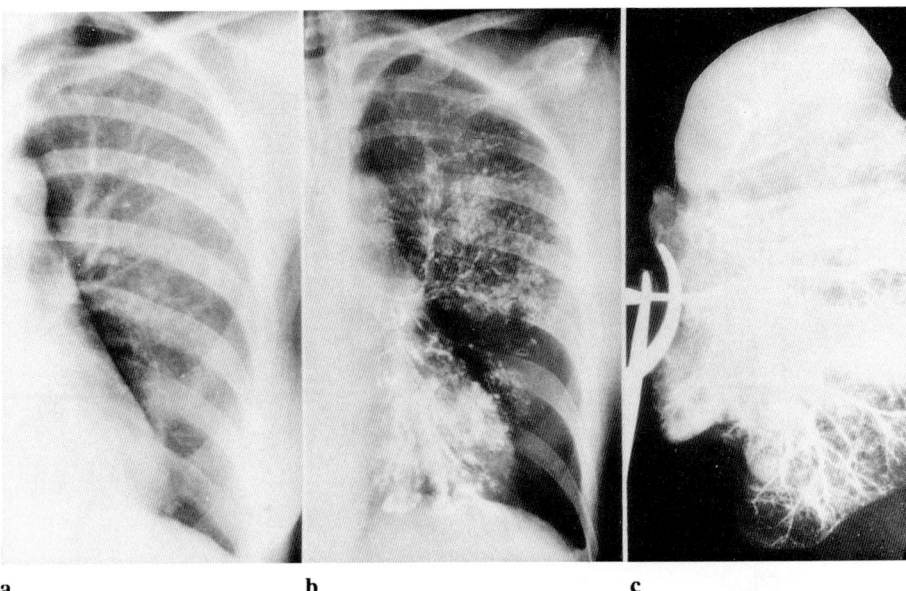

a              b               c

**Fig. 44a–c.** Hyperlucency as an expression of bronchiectasis. Localized hyperlucency of the left lower lobe due to Swyer-James syndrome. **a** Close-up of the left lung where one can see the reduction of the vascularity of the lower half of the left lung. **b** Close-up of the left lung showing extensive bronchiectasis involving the left lower lobe. **c** Specimen radiograph of the resected left lower lobe where one can observe the patent pulmonary arteries. The hyperlucency was due to air-trapping from collapsible bronchiectasis of the lower lobe of the left lung (Swyer-James syndrome)

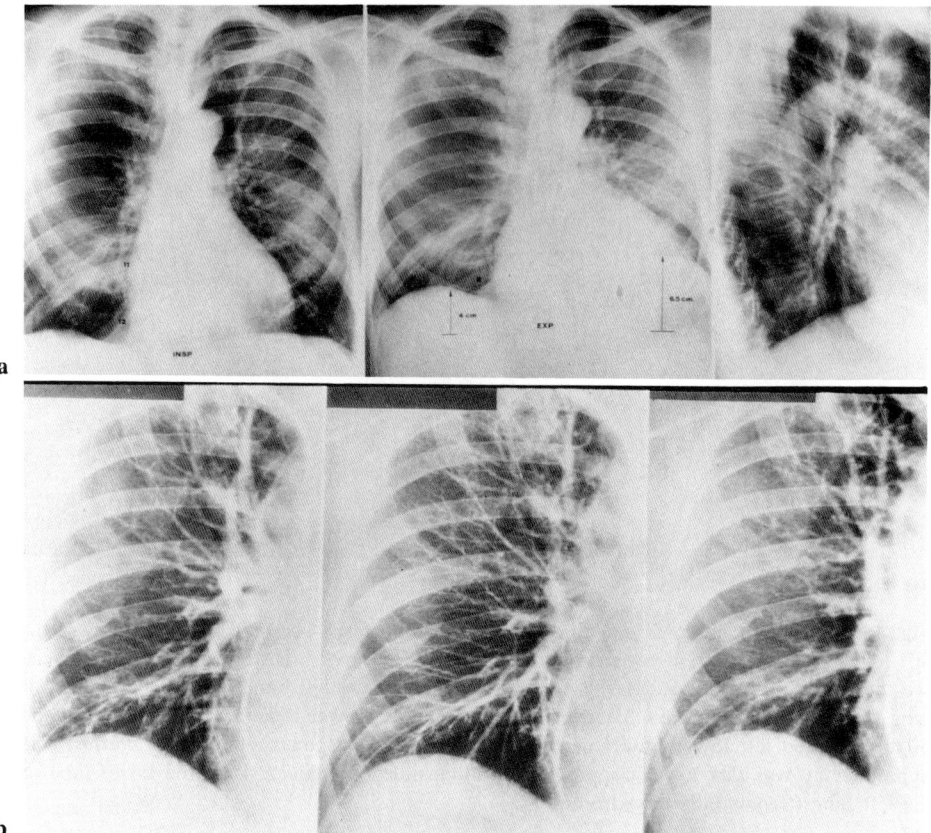

a

b

**Fig. 45a–e.** Another example of hyperlucency due to Swyer-James syndrome. **a** The right mid-lung field (*left*) showed localized hyperlucency, and evidence of air-trapping was observed in the radiograph of the expiratory phase (*middle*). Note that the left hemidiaphragm rose more than the right. A right lateral view chest radiograph (*right*) was normal. **b** Selective right pulmonary arteriograms (*left, middle, right*) showing a reduction in caliber and number of pulmonary arteries in the right mid-lung field. **c** Selective right bronchial arteriogram. There was enlargement of the bronchial arteries and bronchial hypervascularity suggestive of an inflammatory process. **d, e** Bronchographic examination revealed cylindrical bronchiectasis which collapsed during expiration at the time of cinebronchography. Air-trapping explained the focal hyperlucency observed on the plain film of the chest. When localized hyperlucency is found, one should consider bronchopulmonary disease and vascular insufficiency, after ruling out technical errors and absence of soft tissues of the ipsilateral hemithorax. Fluoroscopy and/or expiratory films should exclude the former. Perfusion pulmonary scan and arteriography will diagnose the latter

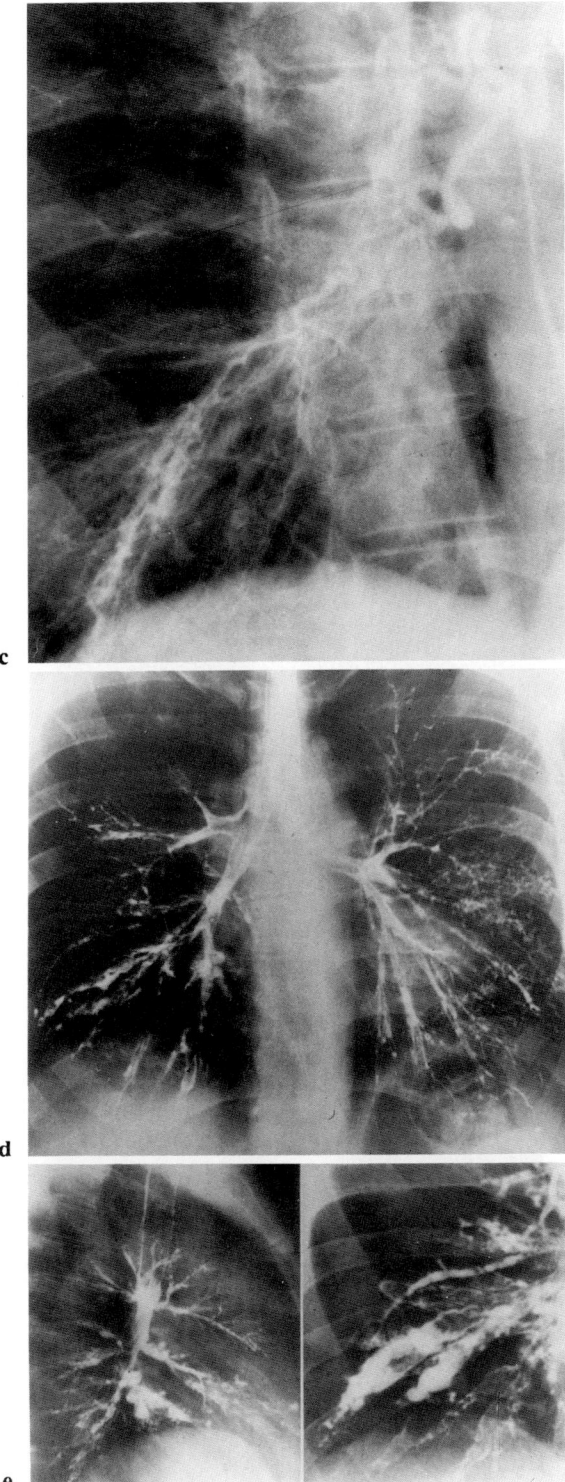

c

d

e

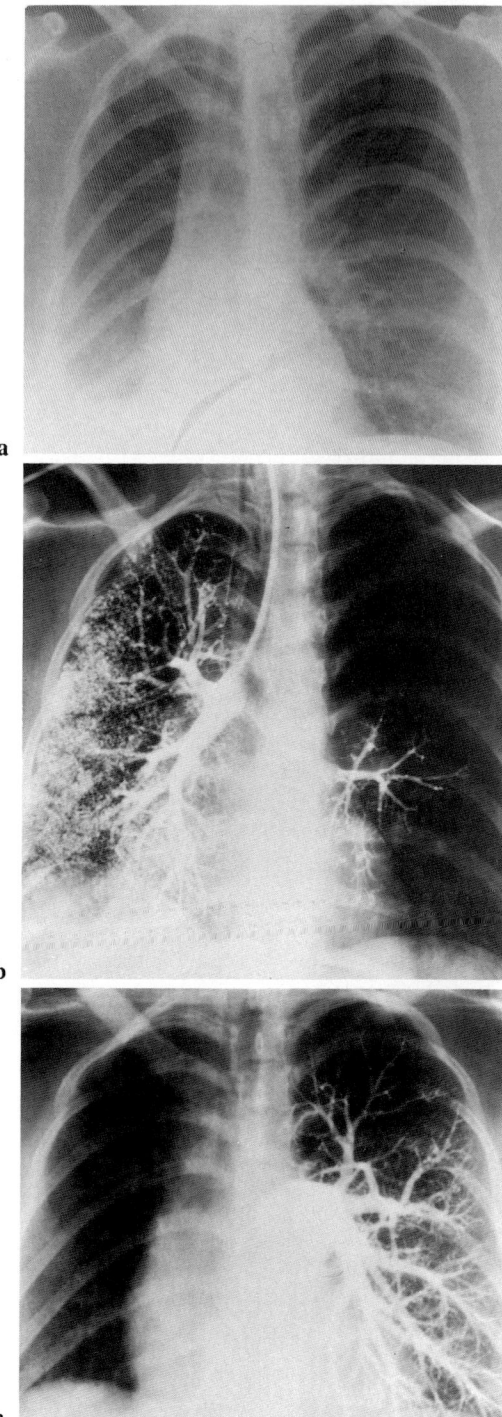

a

b

c

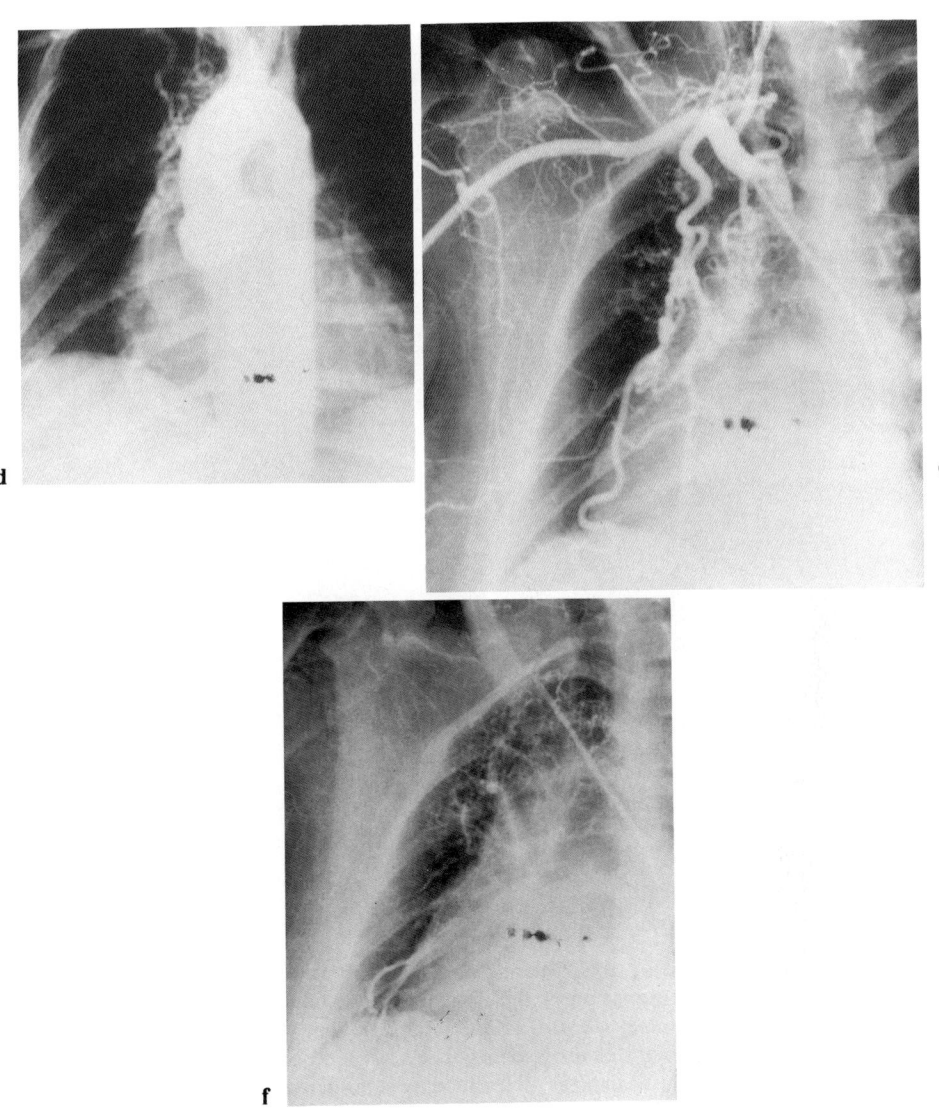

d

e

f

**Fig. 46a–f.** Hyperlucency due to vascular insufficiency. Agenesis of the right pulmonary artery causing localized hyperlucency of the right lung. **a** Frontal view radiograph showing internal thoracic asymmetry characterized by reduction in volume of the right hemithorax, shift of the mediastinum to the right, and paucity of the pulmonary vasculature. Differential diagnosis would include pulmonary arterial insufficiency, emphysema, or air-trapping from Swyer-James syndrome. **b** Selective bronchogram shows normal bronchial tree. This excludes the Swyer-James syndrome. The bronchogram was an unnecessary study. **c** Pulmonary arteriogram shows agenesis of the right pulmonary artery. **d–f** Arterial studies. Note increased arterial hypervascularity arising from the bronchial arteries and right internal mammary artery

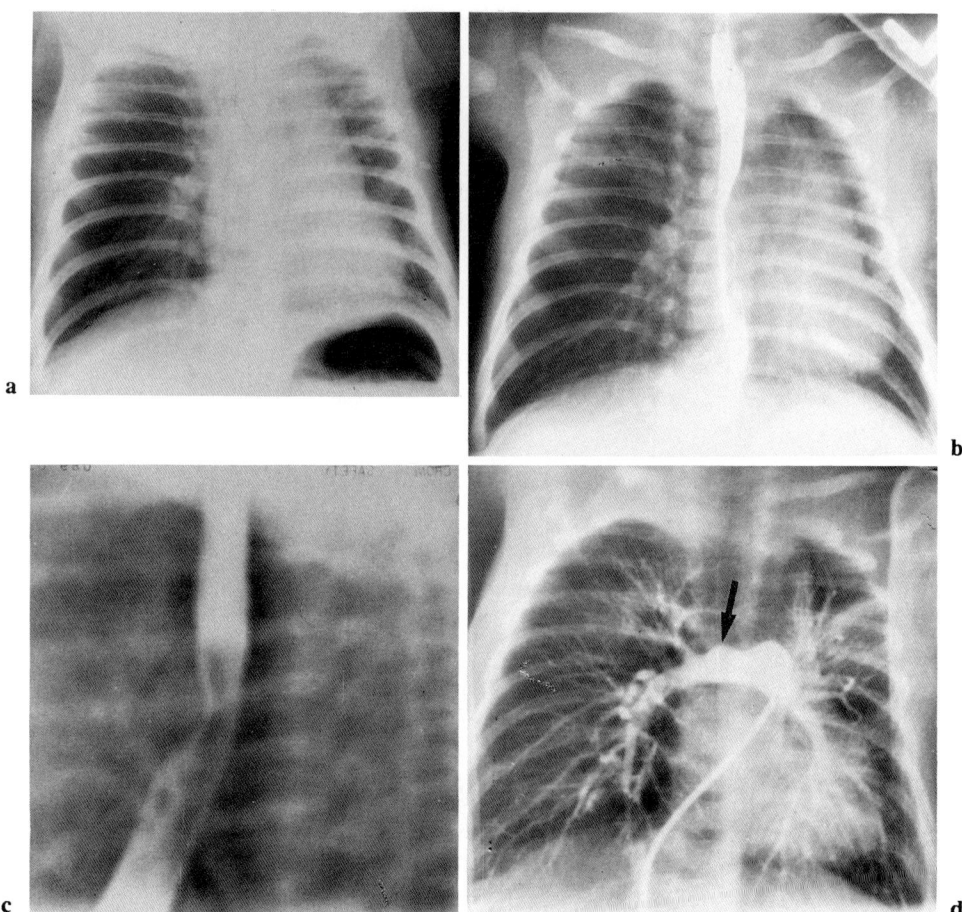

a

b

c

d

Fig. 47a–g. Pulmonary artery sling causing unilateral hyperlucency. a Frontal view chest radiograph showing hyperexpansion of the right lung and shift of the mediastinum to the left. This patient had *inspiratory wheezes* affecting the right lung. b Barium swallow showing discrete narrowing of the mid-thoracic esophagus. c Lateral esophagogram showing anterior indentation of mid-thoracic esophagus. d Pulmonary arteriogram. Frontal projection. Note a convex density above right pulmonary artery (*arrow*). e Lateral view of a pulmonary arteriogram. Note abnormal course of the left pulmonary artery which crossed in front of the thoracic esophagus, arose from the pulmonary trunk, coursed above the right mainstem bronchus, and traversed the mediastinum from right to left interposed between the trachea and the esophagus. f Bronchogram showing smooth narrowing of the proximal right mainstem bronchus (*arrow*) which proved to be related to the pulmonary artery sling. g Diagrammatic representation of a pulmonary artery sling

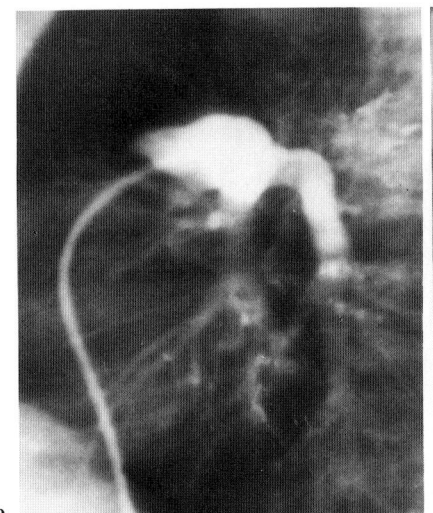

e

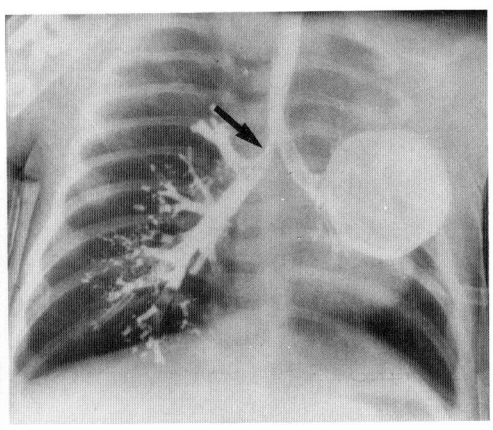

f

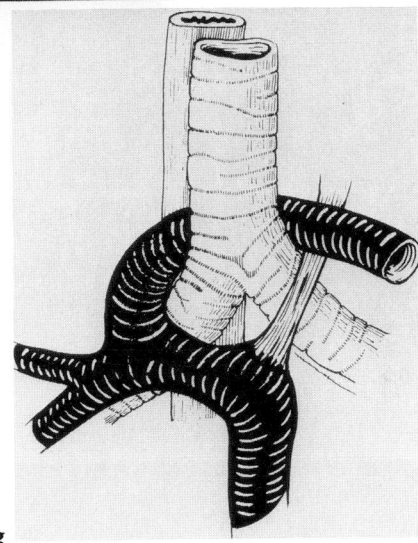

g

70

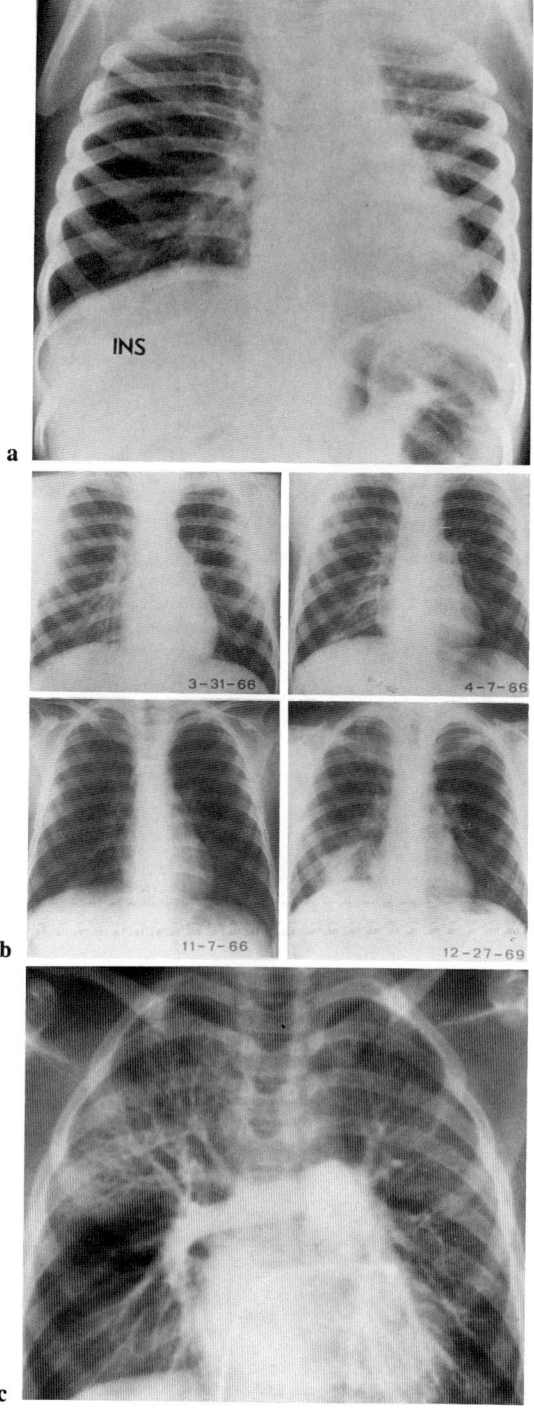

INS

3-31-66

4-7-66

11-7-66

12-27-69

a

b

c

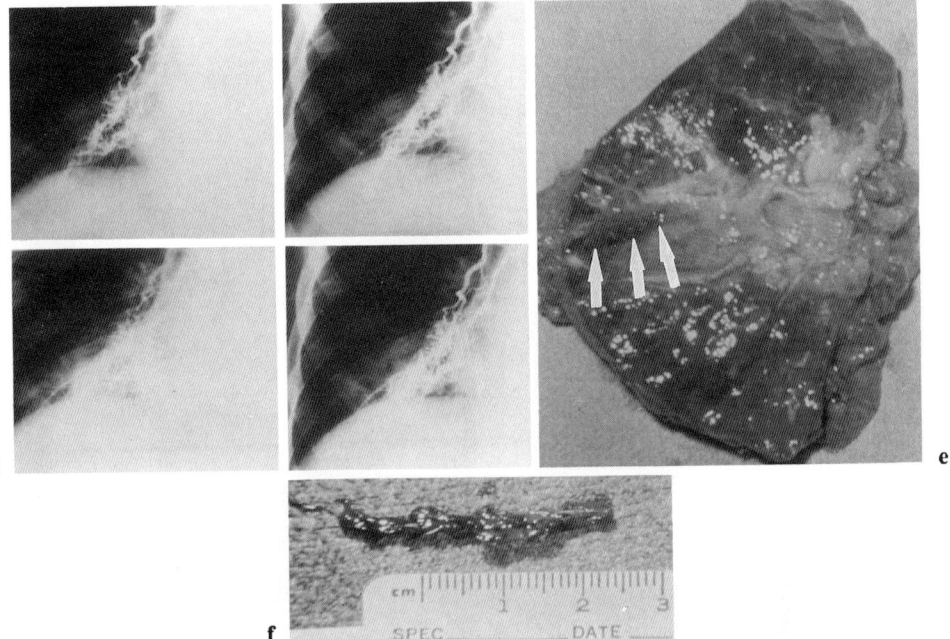

**Fig. 48a–f.** Focal hyperlucency due to occult foreign body. **a** Frontal view radiograph showing hyperlucency of lower half of the right lung. **b** Sequential chest radiographs which revealed intermittent episodes of pneumonia affecting the right lower lobe. The patient presented with "asthma hemoptysis" and recurrent pulmonary infection. **c** Pulmonary arteriogram showing paucity of the pulmonary vasculature in the lower half of the right lung. **d** Selective bronchial arteriograms revealed increased bronchial hypervascularity suggesting an inflammatory process to be present in the right lower lobe. **e** Specimen removed revealing a foreign body in the right main bronchus (*arrows*). **f** The foreign body proved to be a piece of a pine tree. Whenever wheezing is present in a patient with hemoptysis and recurrent pulmonary pathology, an occult foreign body should be suspected and the patient should undergo bronchoscopy and bronchography

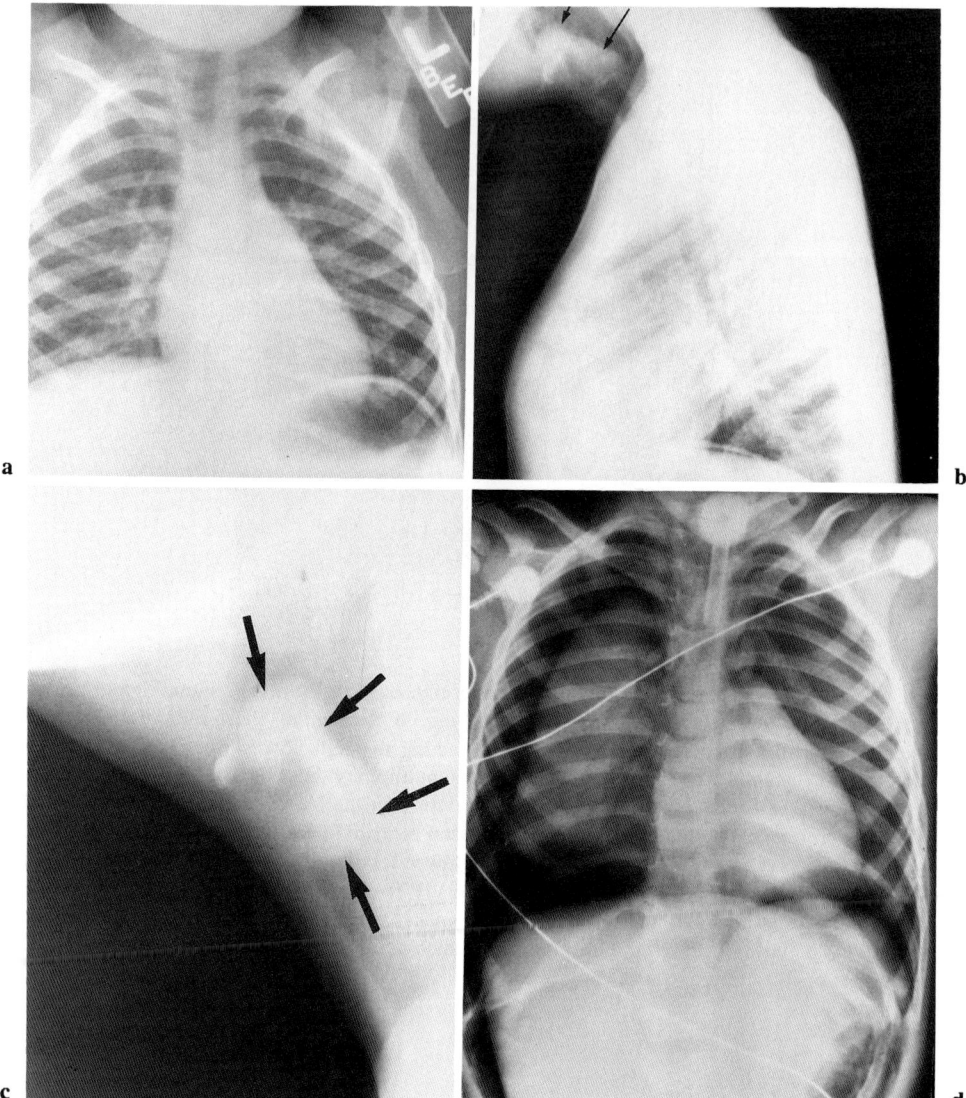

a

b

c

d

**Fig. 49a–d.** Importance of correct examination of the upper airways. Infant with considerable breathing difficulty. **a** Frontal view chest radiograph interpreted correctly as negative. **b** Lateral view of the chest showed a mass at the level of the larynx (*arrows*). **c** Close-up of the larynx showing a mass (*arrows*) which represented epiglottitis. **d** Patient underwent a traumatic intubation and as a result pneumothorax, pneumomediastinum, and pneumoperitoneum developed. The patient survived all these complications uneventfully

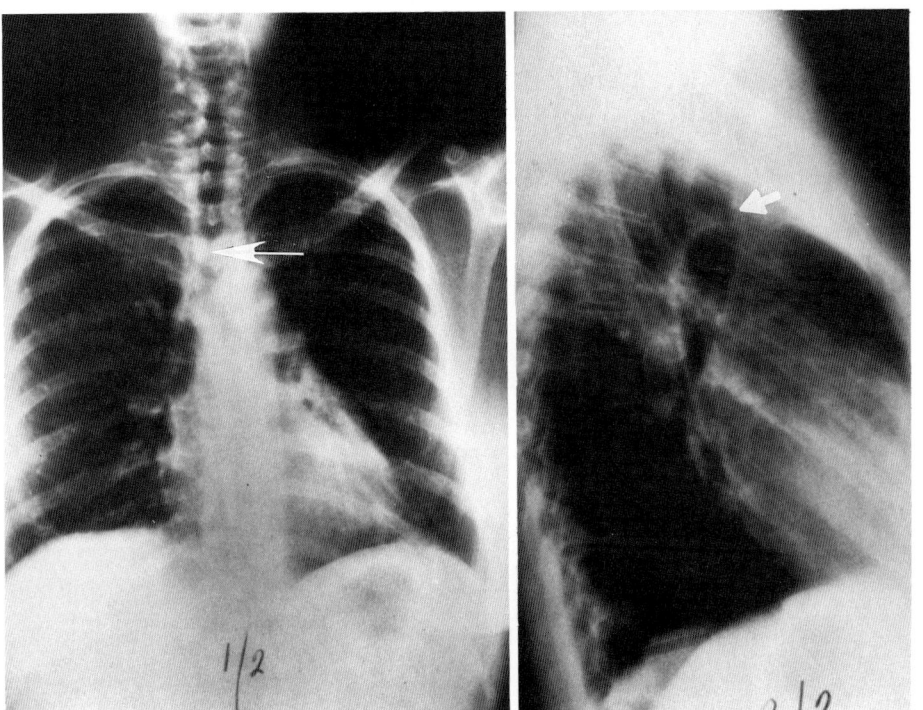

a                                                                                    b

**Fig. 50a, b.** Importance of correct examination of the upper airways. Tracheal stenosis secondary to prolonged intubation. **a, b** Frontal and lateral view chest radiographs showed focal tracheal stenosis (*arrows*). Patient had difficulty breathing and the heart and lungs appeared radiographically unremarkable. Whenever a patient presents with dyspnea and there are no cardiac, pulmonary, neurologic or hematologic reasons to explain the dyspnea, one should pay careful attention to the proximal airway: larynx, trachea and proximal bronchi

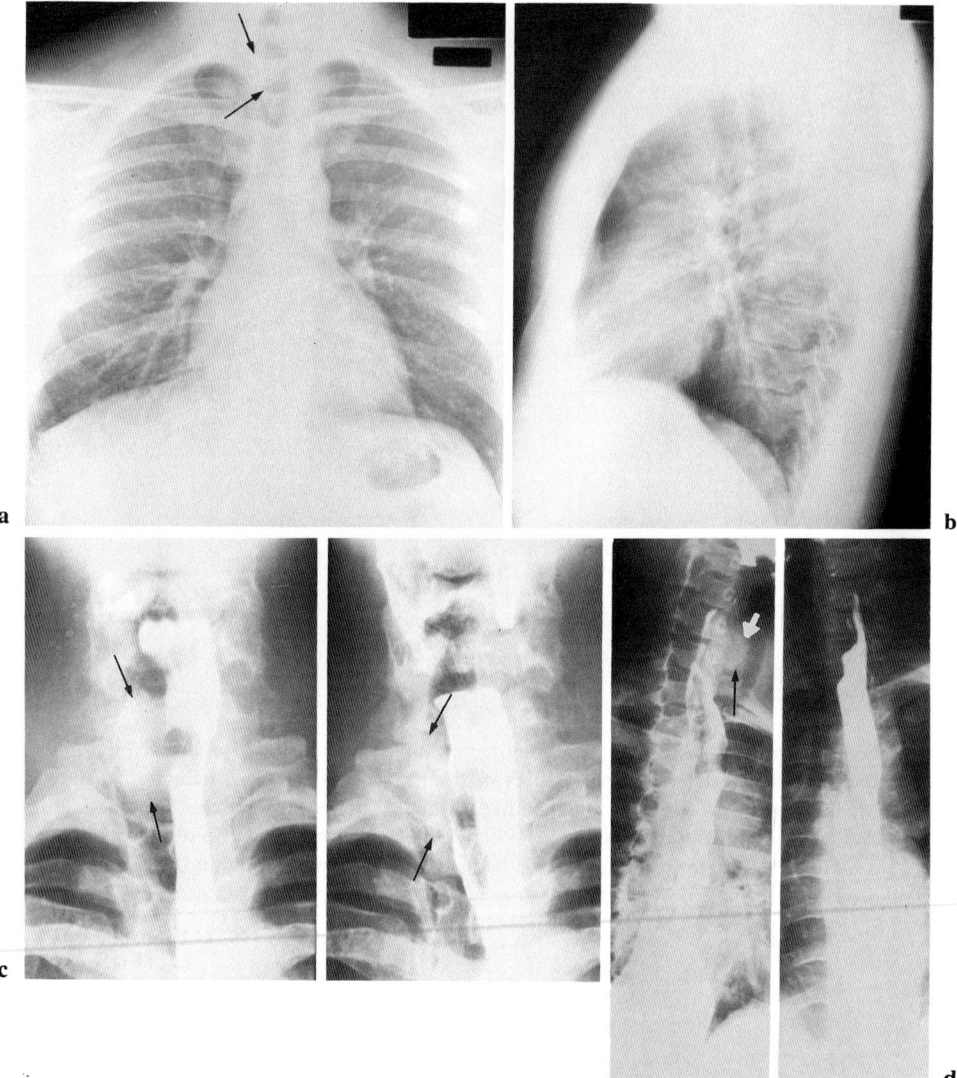

**Fig. 51a–f.** Importance of correct examination of the upper airways. Primary carcinoma of the trachea in a 28-year-old man. **a, b** Frontal and lateral view chest radiographs taken in a country in Central America and interpreted as negative. In the frontal view, the right wall of the trachea appeared indistinct (*arrows*). The patient had difficulty breathing and swallowing. **c** Barium swallow showing a mass in the esophagus and a larger mass occupying the lumen of the right side of the trachea (*arrows*). **d** Barium swallow revealed again the mass between the esophagus and the trachea (*arrows*). **e** CT of pharynx showed large retrotracheal mass which proved to represent a primary tracheal carcinoma. **f** Specimen showing large tumor affecting the upper trachea

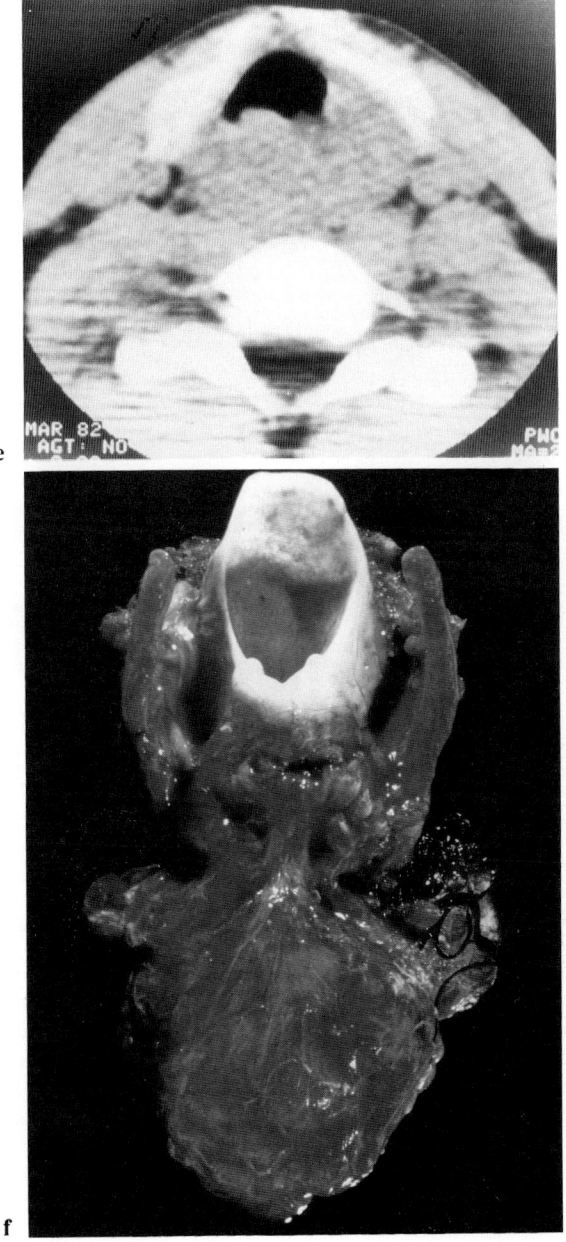

e

f

76

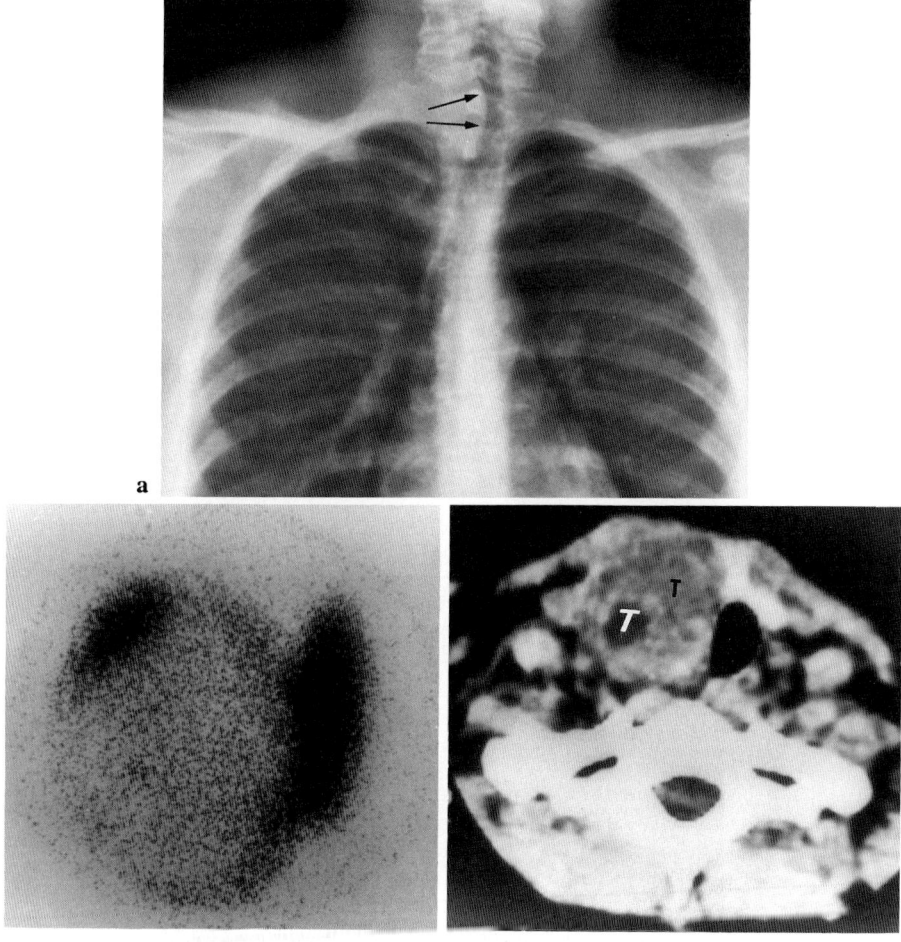

**Fig. 52a–c.** Importance of correct examination of the upper airways. Carcinoma of the thyroid gland. **a** Frontal view chest radiograph interpreted as negative by an internist. Note compression and displacement of the trachea to the left (*arrows*). **b** Scintigram showing photopenic mass involving the right lobe of the thyroid gland. **c** CT examination showing mass (*black T*) wrapped around the trachea (*white T*). This proved to be a papillary carcinoma of the trachea. Thyroid masses are commonly missed by nonradiologists (and "harried" radiologists!)

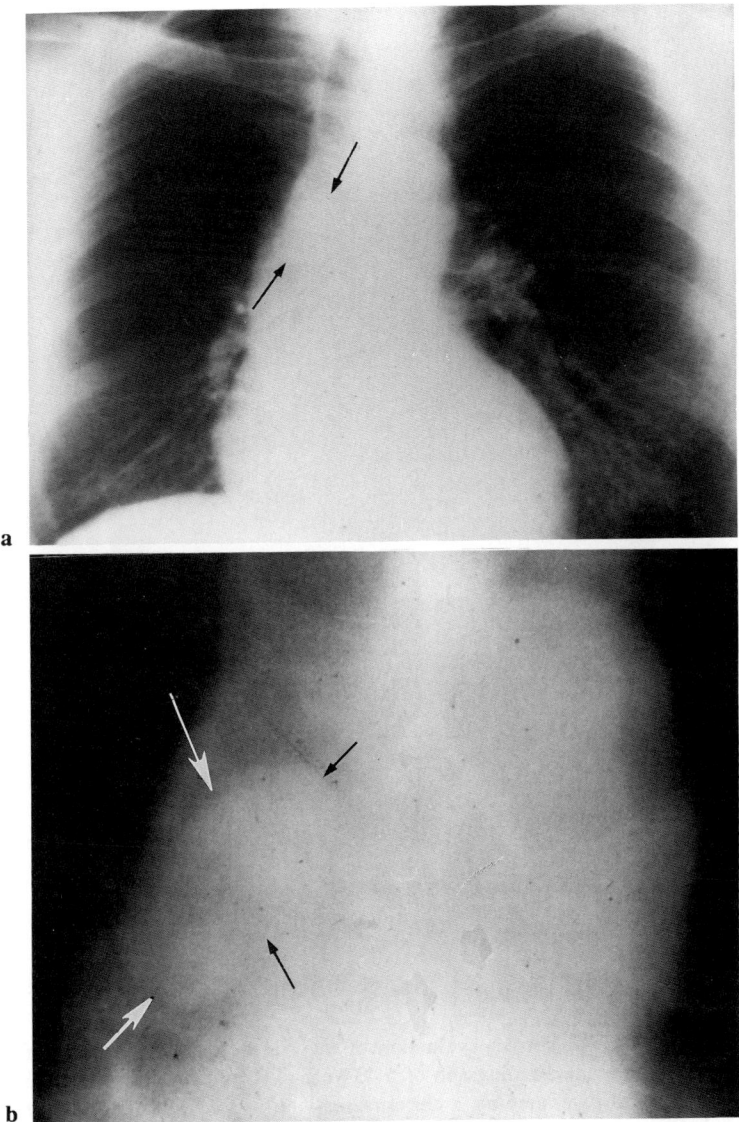

**Fig. 53a, b.** Importance of correct assessment of the upper airways. Bronchial carcinoid. **a** Overexposed frontal view radiograph taken in an internist's office. A mass was seen occupying the lumen of the right mainstem bronchus (*arrows*). This patient presented with hemoptysis. **b** Close-up of this region showing an olive-sized mass (*arrows*) which proved to be a bronchial carcinoid

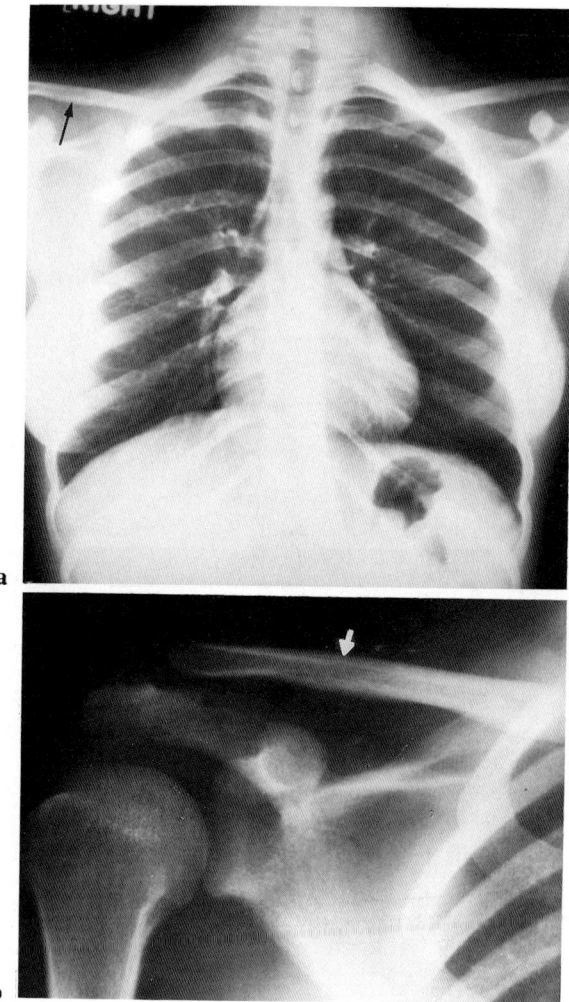

**Fig. 54a, b.** Importance of correct evaluation of the bones. Ewing's sarcoma of the right clavicle. **a** Frontal view chest radiograph of a 23-year-old woman who complained of right shoulder pain. She was examined by a chiropractor who missed a lesion of the right clavicle (*arrow*). **b** Close-up of the right clavicle. Note permeative destructive pattern (*arrow*), which, on biopsy, proved to represent a Ewing's sarcoma. Where there is a palpable mass or persistent shoulder pain, a radiographic examination of the shoulder and of the cervical spine may reveal unsuspected bone pathology

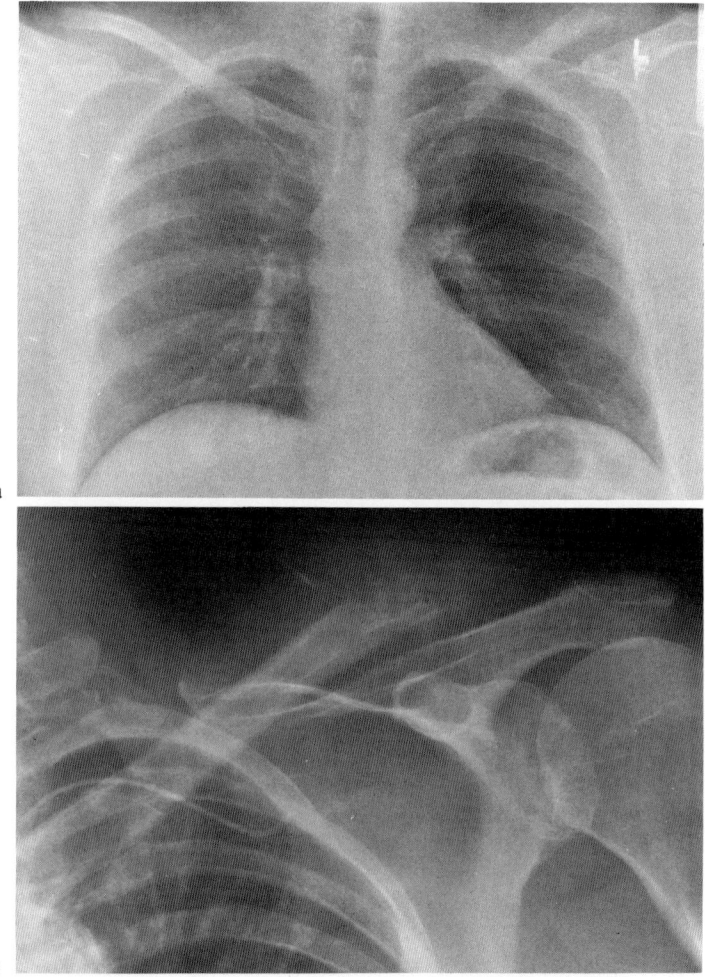

**Fig. 55a, b.** Importance of correct evaluation of the bones. Ewing's sarcoma of the left clavicle. **a** The frontal view chest radiograph showed ill-defined left outer clavicle. The patient complained of shoulder pain and was diagnosed as having bursitis. **b** Close-up of the left clavicle showing destructive changes

80

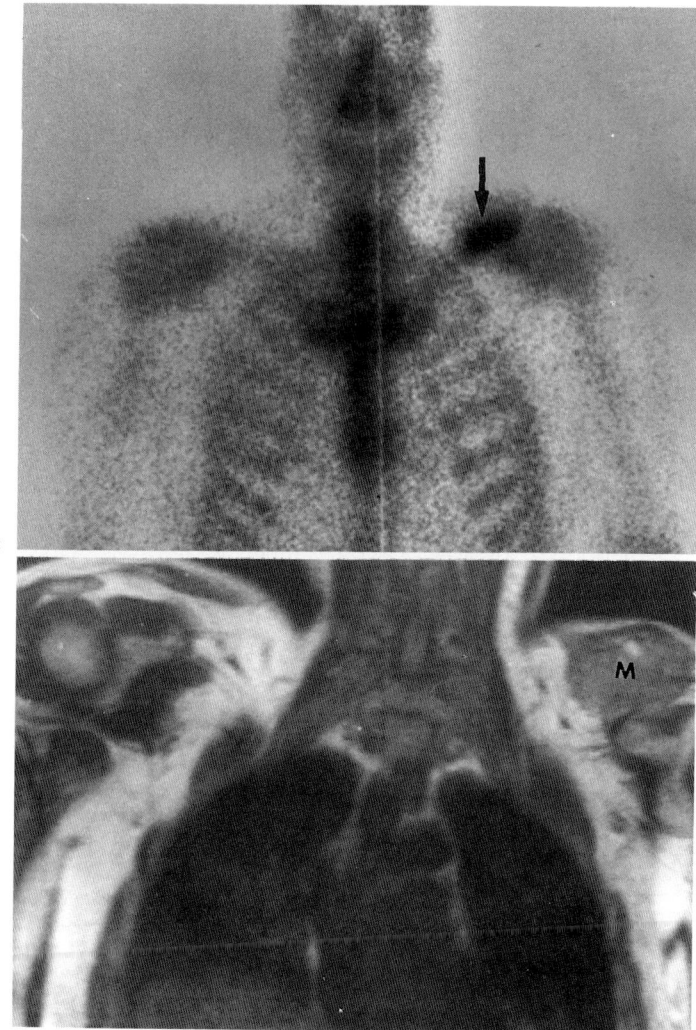

c

d

**Fig. 55c, d.** Importance of correct evaluation of the bones. Ewing's carcinoma of the left clavicle. **c** Bone scan showed increased activity at the level of the left clavicle and supra-clavicular region (*arrow*). **d** MRI revealed a mass (*M*) extending into the left supraclavicular fossa which proved to be a Ewing's sarcoma

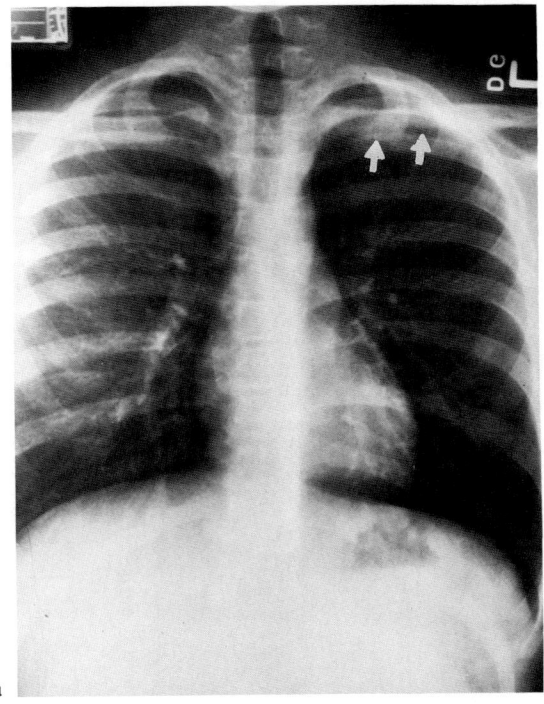

a

**Fig. 56a.** Importance of correct evaluation of the bones. Chronic osteomyelitis of the left clavicle. Frontal view chest radiograph interpreted as negative. Note poorly defined medial aspect of the left clavicle (*arrows*)

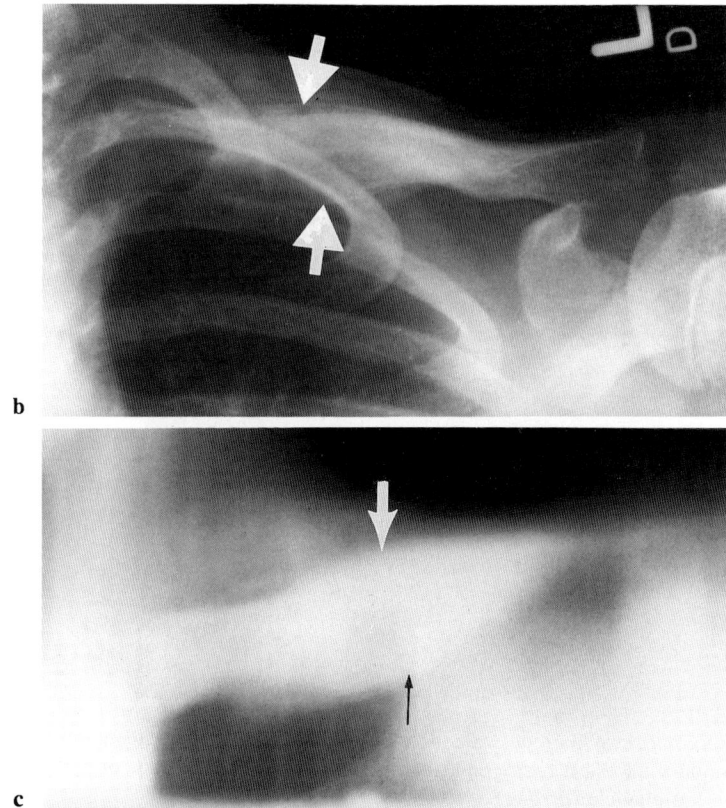

b

c

**Fig. 56b, c.** Importance of correct evaluation of the bones. **b** Close-up of the left clavicle showed sclerosis of the mid-clavicle and focal destructive changes (*arrows*). **c** Tomogram of the left clavicle showing marked sclerosis (*arrows*). This proved, on biopsy, to be chronic osteomyelitis

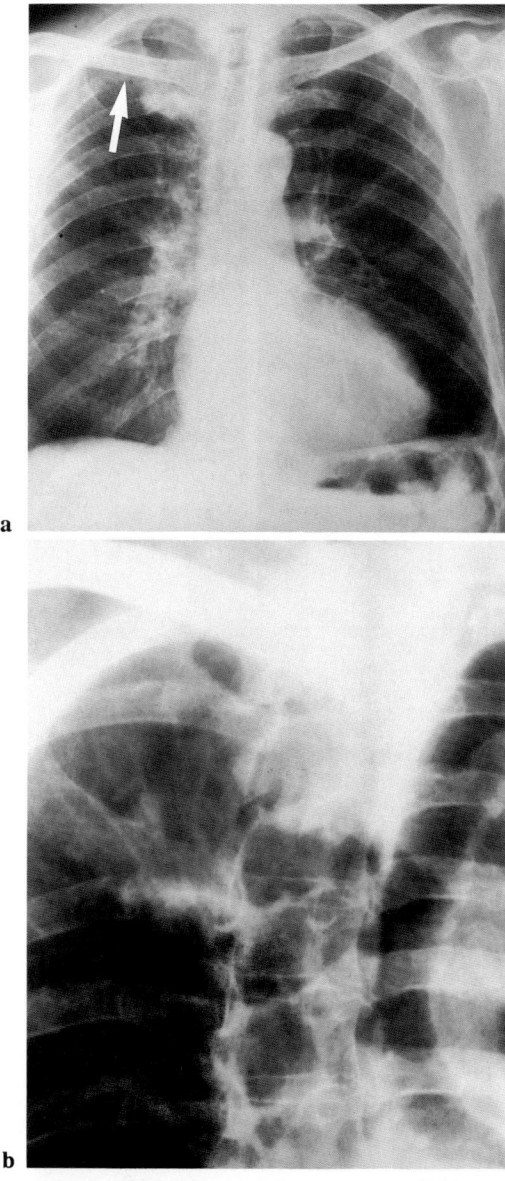

**Fig. 57a, b.** Importance of correct examination of bones. Rib destroyed by metastatic bronchogenic carcinoma. **a** Frontal view chest radiograph interpreted as negative. Note absent posterior arch of the right third rib (*arrow*). **b** Oblique view showed destruction of the posterior arch of the right third rib

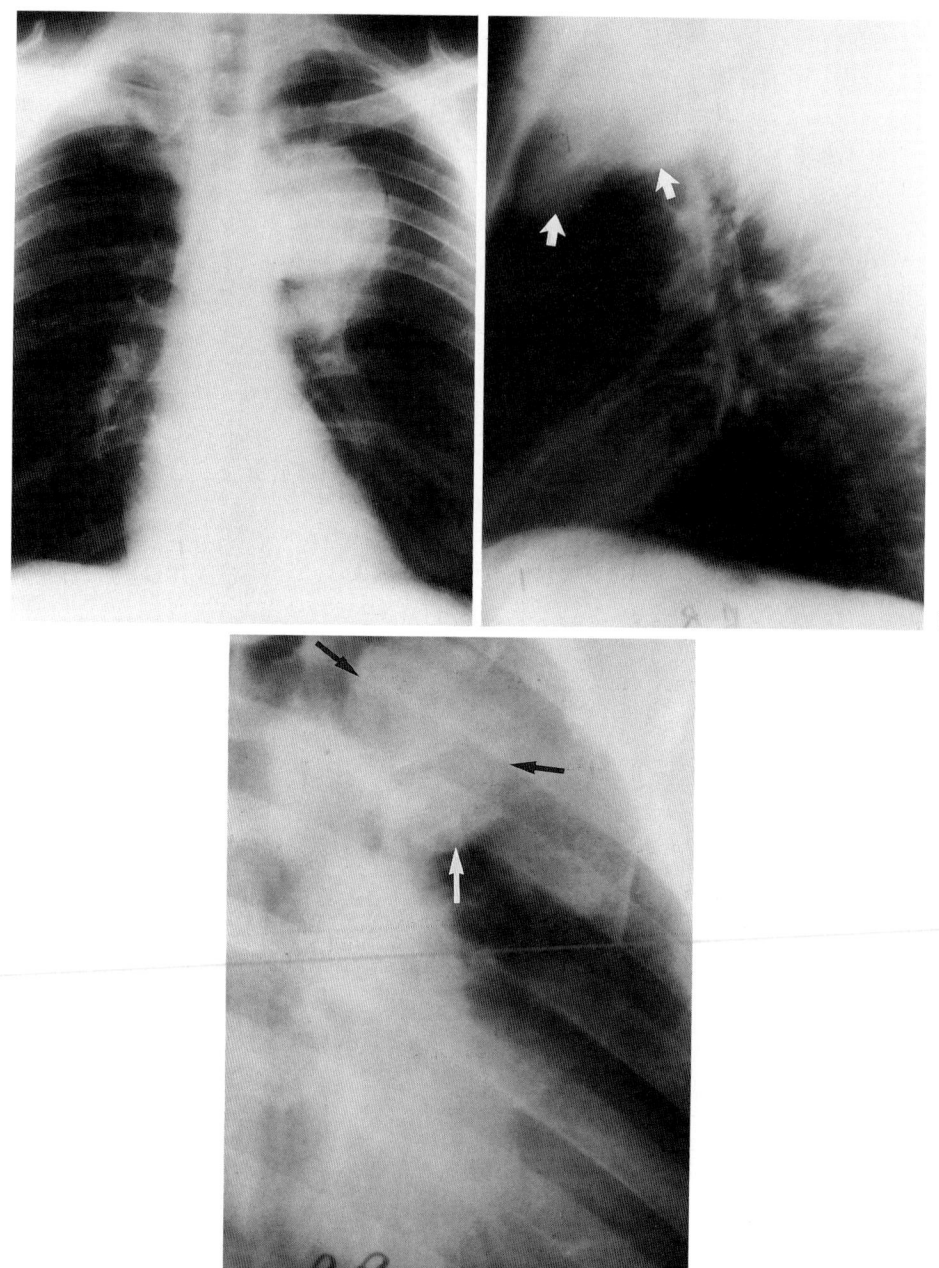

a

b

c

**Fig. 58a–c.** Importance of correct examination of bones. Chondrosarcoma of the anterior arch of the left first and second ribs. **a, b** Frontal and lateral view chest radiographs revealing a large mass (*arrows*) which was interpreted as representing a large pulmonary tumor. Note that the relationship of the mass to the rib cage is difficult to establish. **c** Oblique view of the left upper ribs showing that the mass involved the anterior arch of the left first rib (*arrows*). It proved to be a chondrosarcoma

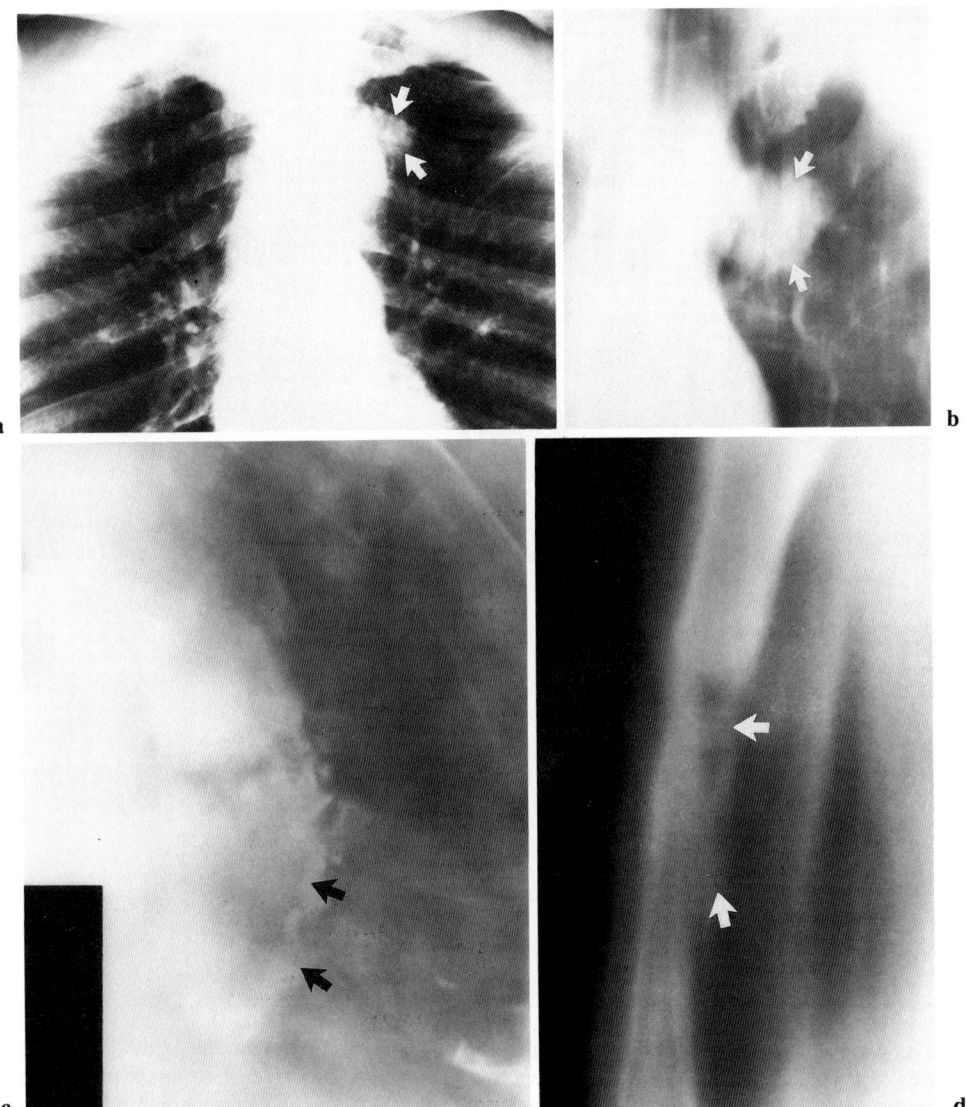

**Fig. 59a–d.** Importance of correct examination of bones. Chondrosarcoma of the sternum, suspected of being a pulmonary neoplasm. **a** Frontal view chest radiograph showing a mass projected close to the aortic knob (*arrows*). **b** Tomogram showing irregular mass which was interpreted as a pulmonary neoplasm (*arrows*). **c, d** Tomograms of the sternum showing destruction of the sternum (*arrows*). The mass represented the intrathoracic extension of a chondrosarcoma of the sternum

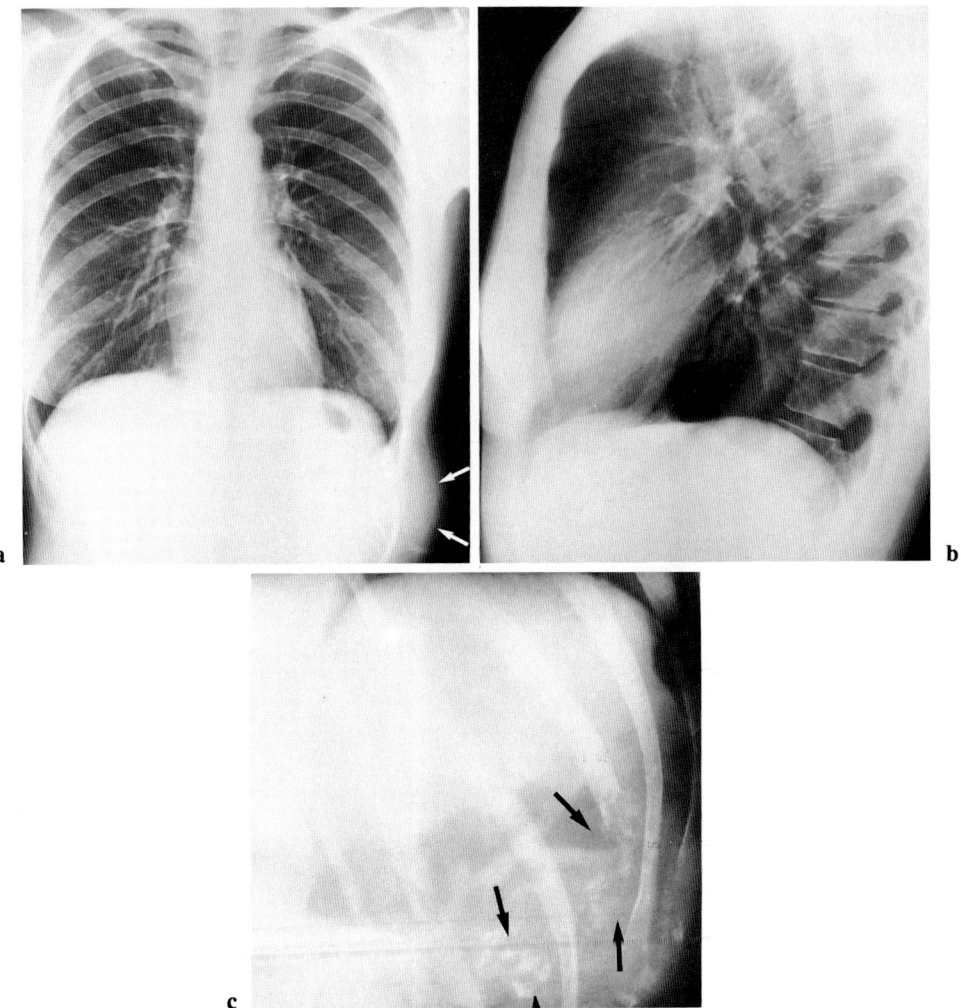

**Fig. 60a–c.** Importance of correct examination of bones. Chondrosarcoma of the left lower ribs. **a** Frontal view chest radiograph reported as negative. However, note mass projecting in the upper portion of the left flank (*arrows*). **b** Lateral view chest radiograph which was negative. **c** Close-up of the left lower ribs showing destruction of the ribs, the mass, and calcifications (*arrows*). The mass proved to be a chondrosarcoma of the rib

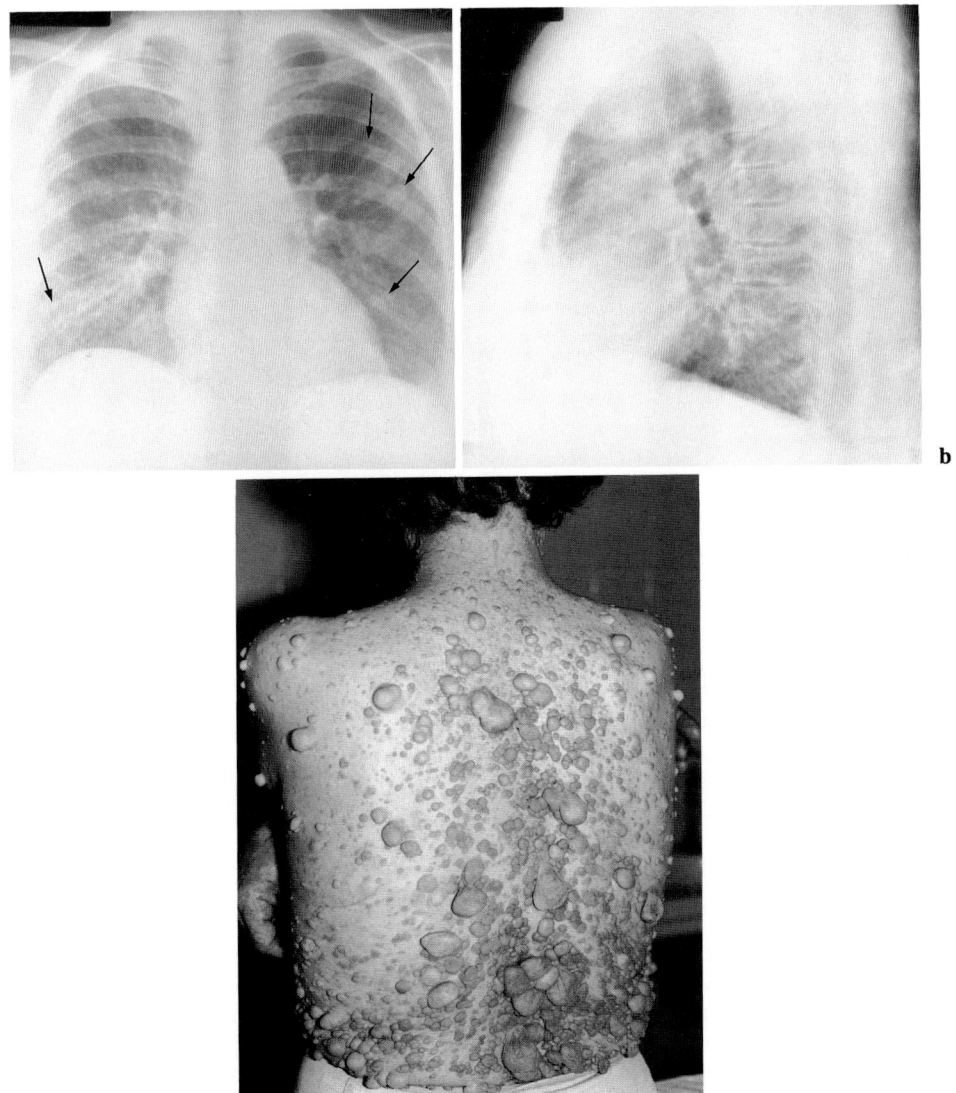

**Fig. 61a–c.** Importance of correct examination of soft tissues. Neurofibromatosis. **a** Frontal view chest radiograph showing multiple nodules diagnosed as being in the lungs (*arrows*). **b** Lateral view chest radiograph. Note that the nodules are in the subcutaneous tissues. **c** Photograph of the patient who had neurofibromatosis. There were no nodules in the lung

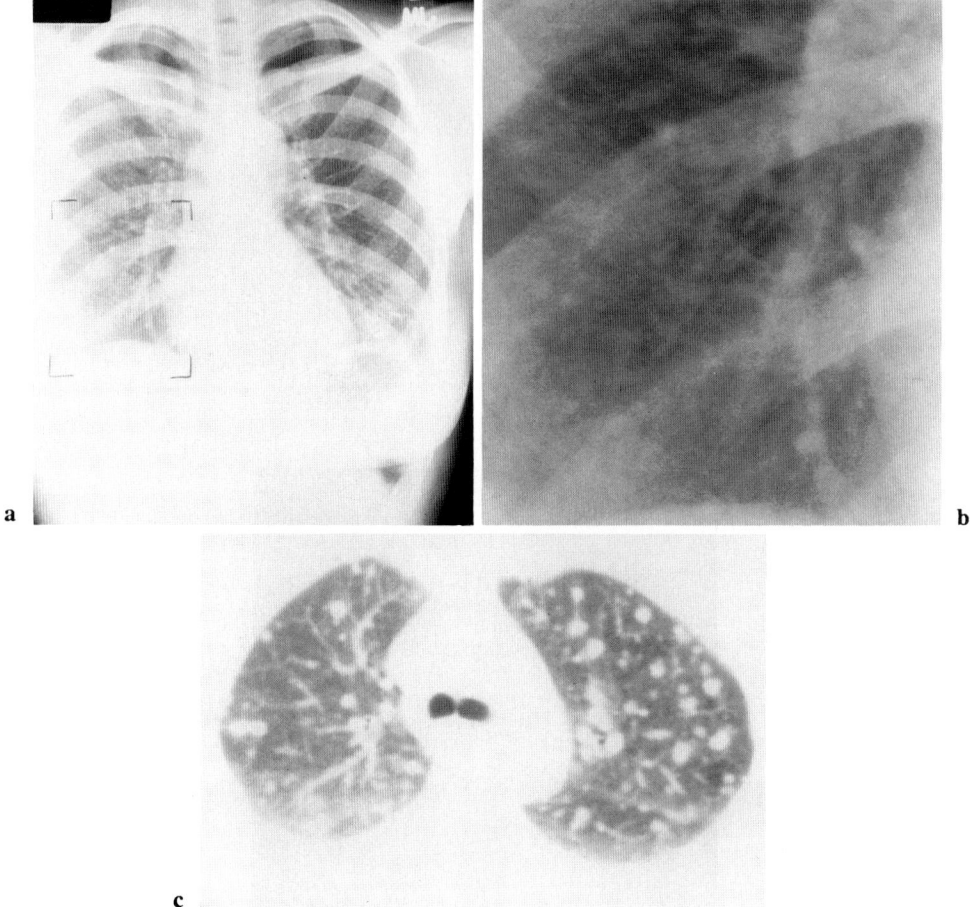

a

b

c

Fig. 62a–f. Importance of correct examination of the soft tissues. Metastatic carcinoma of the breast. a Frontal view chest radiograph showing discrete nodular densities throughout both lungs. b Close-up of the right lung, lower lobe showing multiple discrete pulmonary nodules. c CT examination confirming the presence of bilateral small pulmonary nodules, noncalcified. d CT examination of the chest showing mass in the left breast (*M*). e CT of the chest showing well-circumscribed mass in the left breast, which proved to be a carcinoma (*M*). f Note enlarged left axillary nodes (*arrows*)

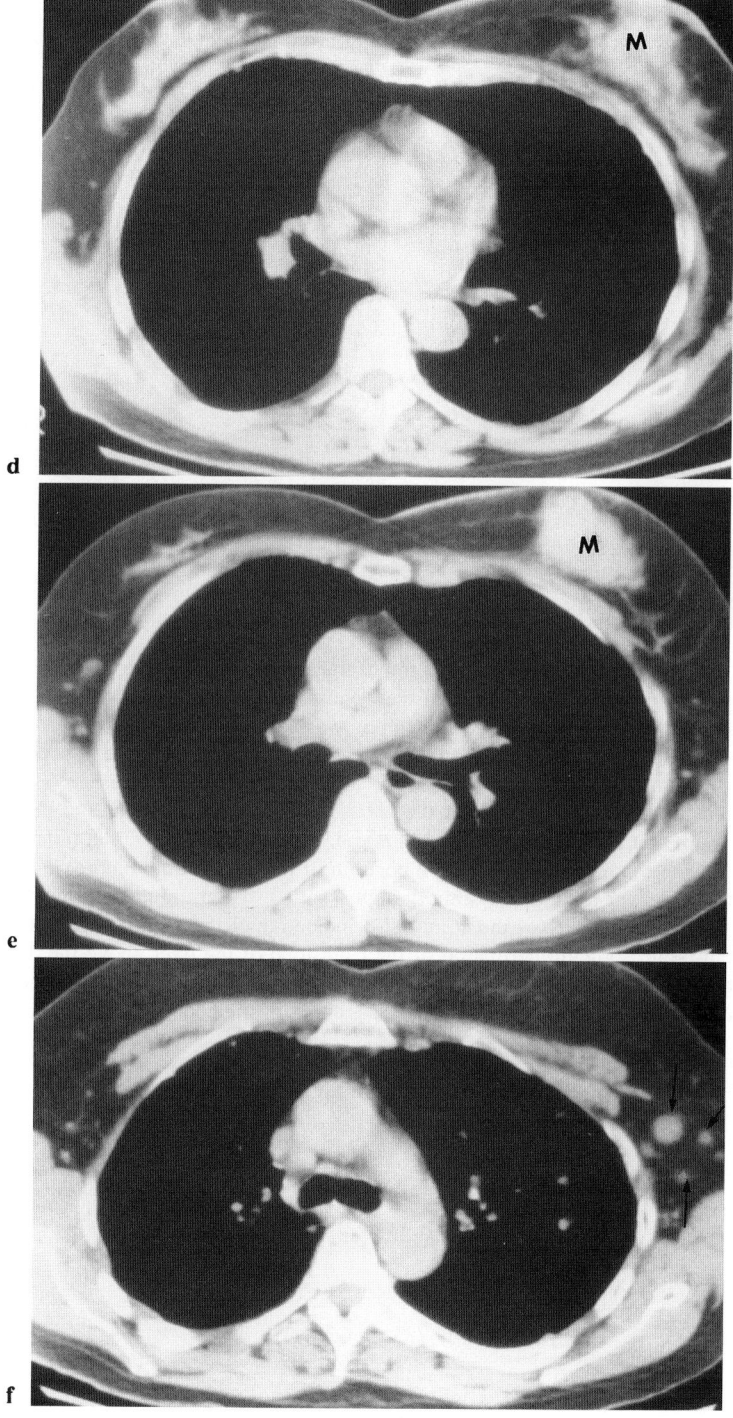

d

e

f

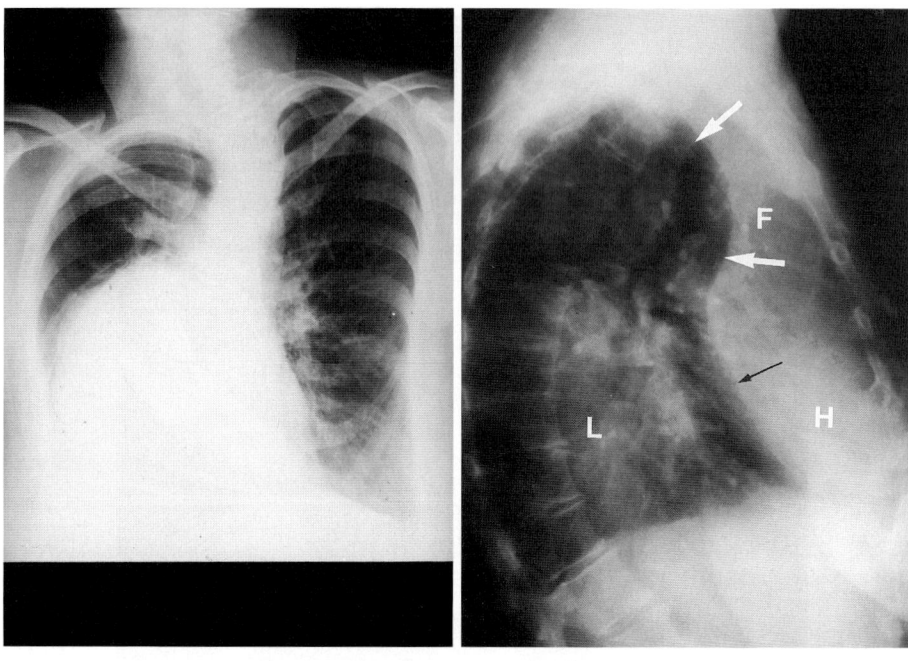

a

b

**Fig. 63a–e.** Importance of correct examination of the abdominal structures. Hypoplastic right lung with herniation of the liver. **a** Frontal view chest radiograph. Note small volume of the right lung and dextroposition of the heart. A mass was seen in the right lower hemithorax. **b** Lateral view chest radiograph. This was a key view for the diagnosis. Note hypoplastic right lung (*arrows*). A mass (*L*) was seen behind the heart (*H*). Fibroadipose tissue (*F*) filled the space between the hypoplastic lung and the anterior chest wall. Note that the only portion of the diaphragm that is visualized is the left dome. **c** Upper gastrointestinal (*GI*) series and small bowel of the same patient. Note high position of the duodenum and proximal jejunum suggesting that the liver is in an abnormally high position. **d** Barium enema showing a high position of the hepatic flexure of the colon, also indicative of the high position of the liver. **e** Hepatic scintigram showing herniation of the right lobe of the liver above the diaphragm. The mass in the chest was not a pulmonary or pleural tumor but the liver. Whenever there is a mass in contact with the diaphragm, the assessment of the abdominal organs is essential

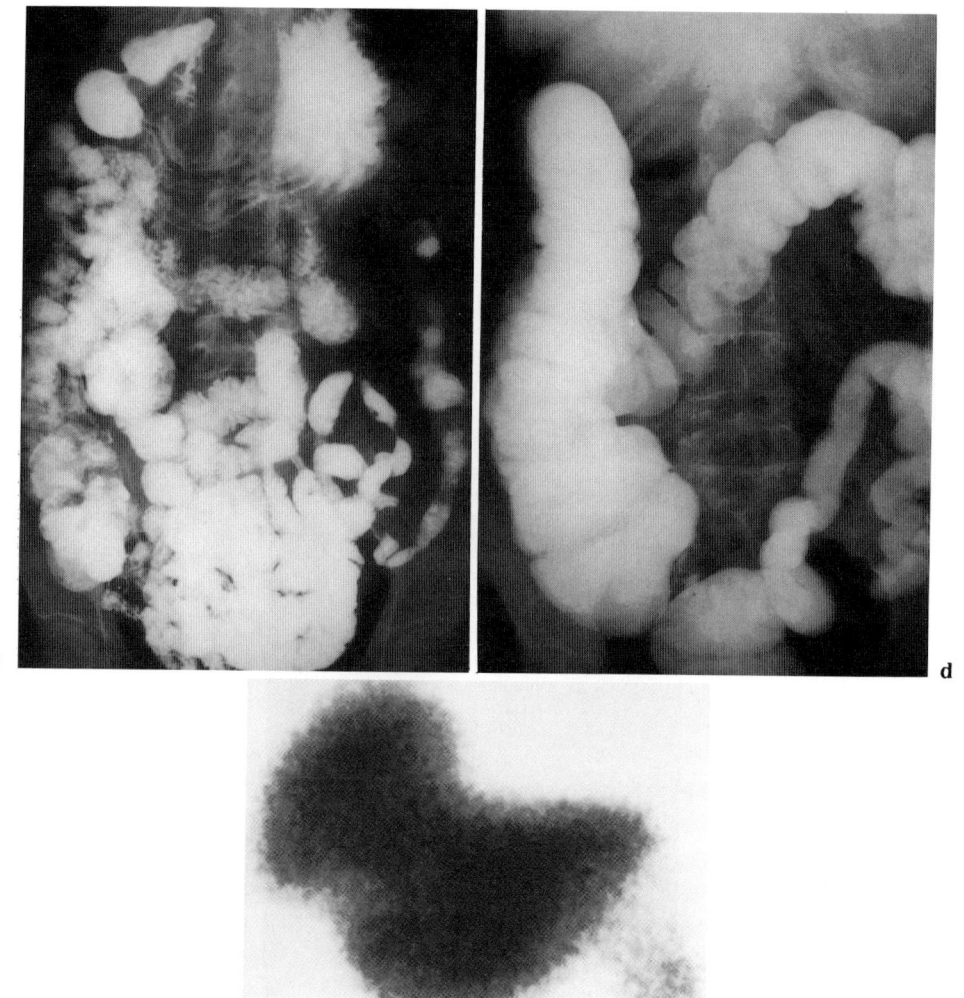

c

d

e

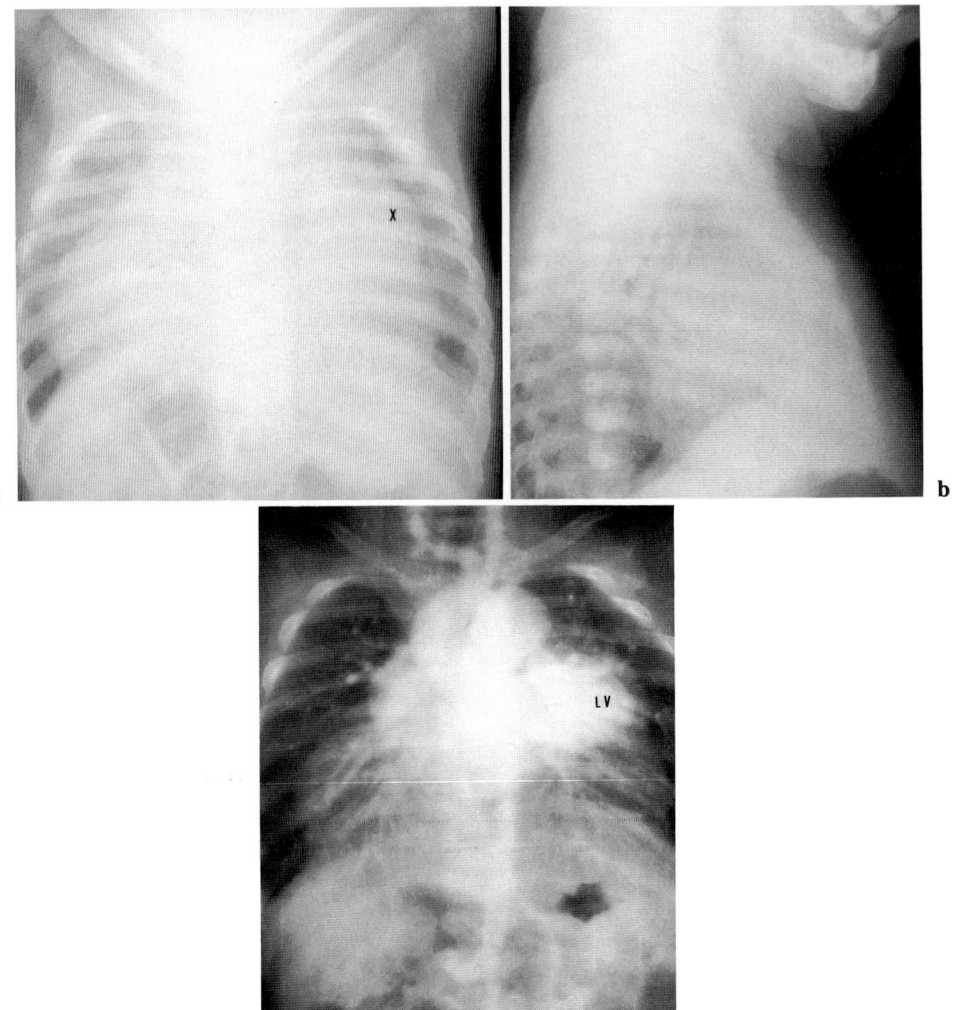

a

b

c

**Fig. 64a–c.** Importance of correct assessment of the abdomen. Liver ectopia. **a** Frontal view chest radiograph showing an apparent situs inversus universalis. Note density under the left dome of the diaphragm which was interpreted as being due to the liver. The heart appeared enlarged. *X* indicates what eventually turned out to be the left ventricle. The patient was admitted for the evaluation of a continuous murmer; a patent ductus arteriosus was suspected. **b** Lateral view which did not contribute any additional information. **c** Angiocardiogram showing that the heart was in the usual position (*LV*, left ventricle). An enlarged pulmonary trunk was noted and simultaneous opacification of the aorta and pulmonary trunk confirmed the presence of a ductus arteriosus. The mass, which was misinterpreted as enlarged heart, represented the liver in the chest which had herniated through a large defect in the tendinous portion of the diaphragm. The patient swallowed air and air was then seen in the fundus of the stomach which was under the left hemidiaphragm. The baby had a scaphoid abdomen which should have suggested the presence of either a congenital diaphragmatic hernia or a high intestinal atresia

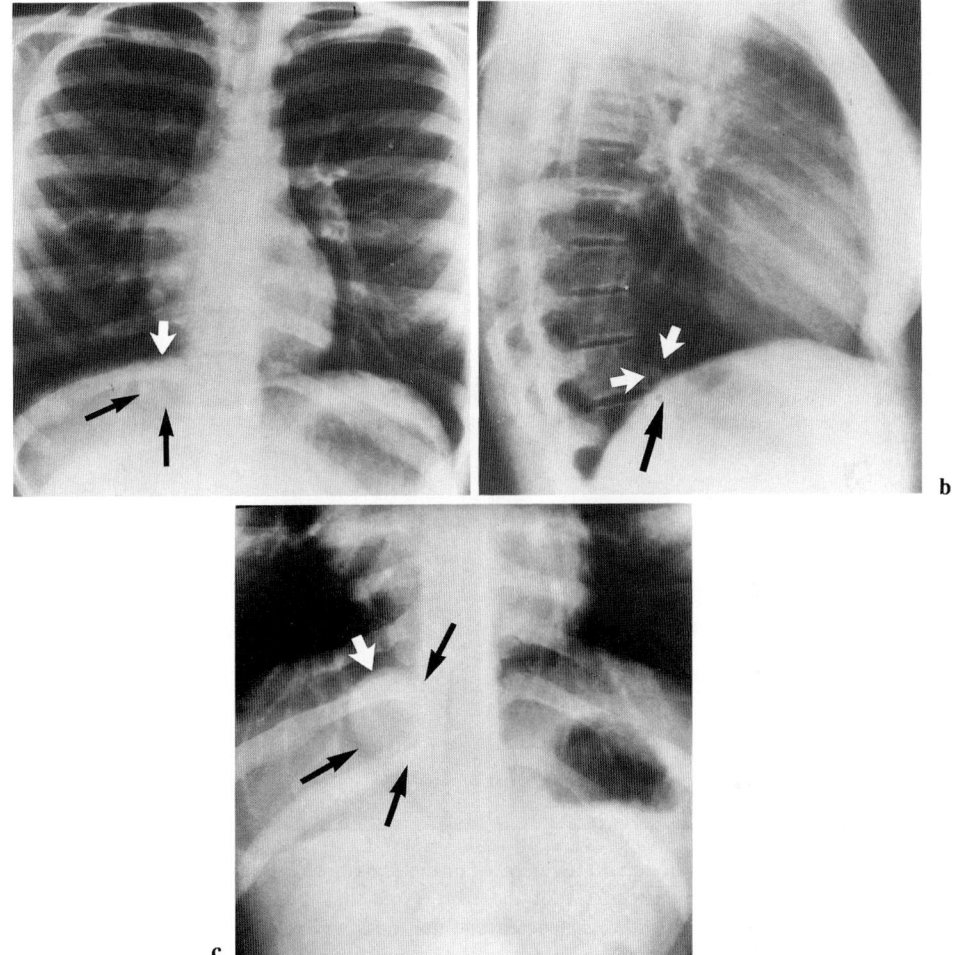

**Fig. 65a–c.** Importance of correct assessment of the abdomen. Intrathoracic accessory liver. **a** Frontal view of an asymptomatic teenager who presented with a mass to the right of the spine (*arrows*). **b** Lateral view chest radiograph faintly showed mass projected at the level of the anterior margin of the lower thoracic spine (*arrows*). **c** A film of the abdomen showed the mass surrounded by air superiorly, medially, and laterally (*arrows*)

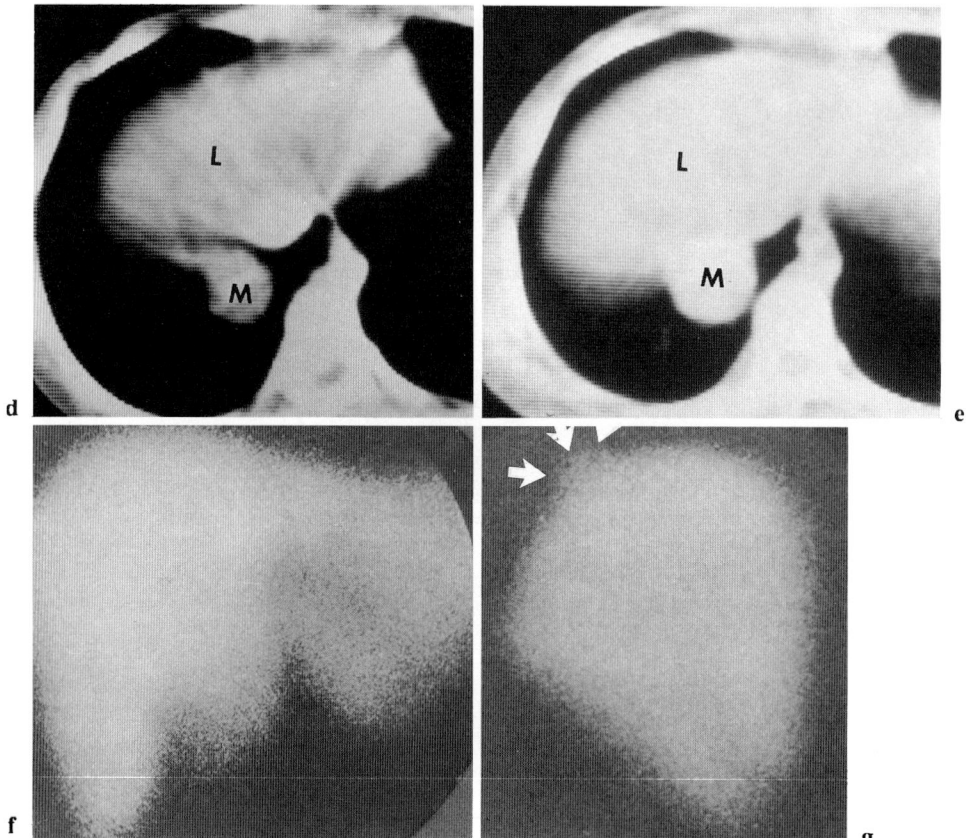

d

e

f

g

Fig. 65d–g. Importance of correct assessment of the abdomen. Intrathoracic accessory liver.
d Nonenhanced and e enhanced CT of the liver. Note that the mass (*M*) had exactly the
same density as the liver (*L*). We suspected that the mass was related to the liver. f Hepatic
scintigram in the frontal projection and g in the lateral projection with the patient upright.
In the frontal projection the liver appeared normal and the mass was not seen. In the lateral projection the mass was seen behind the right lobe of the liver (*arrows*). This was a
pathognomonic finding of an intrathoracic accessory liver

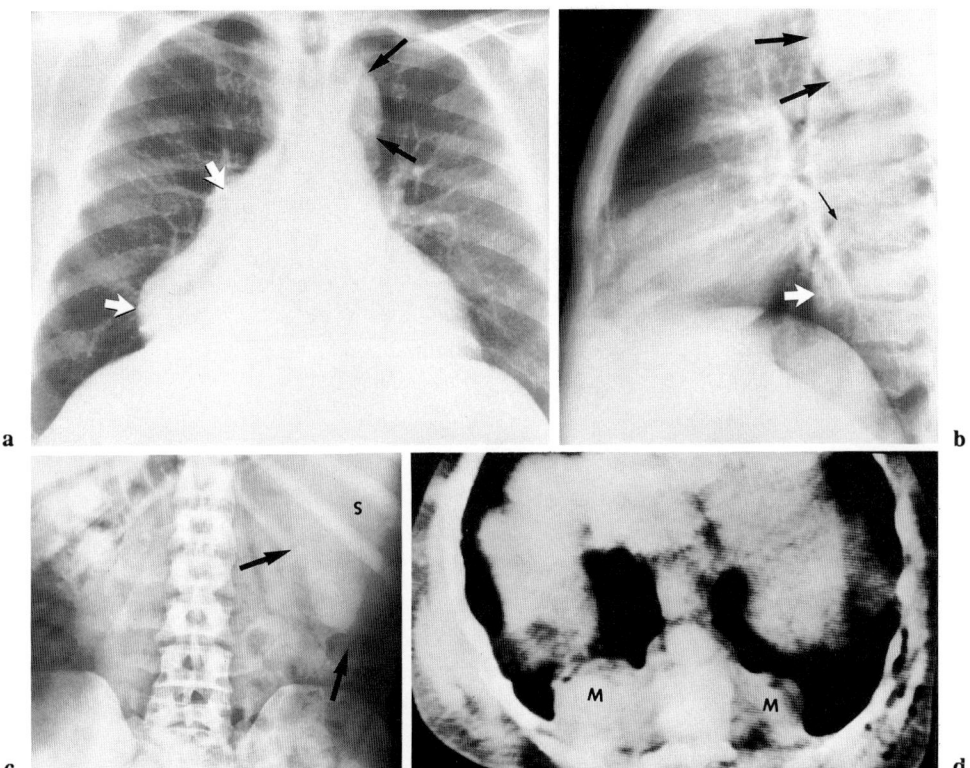

a

b

c

d

**Fig. 66a–d.** Importance of correct assessment of the abdomen. Extramedullary hematopoiesis. **a** Frontal view chest radiograph revealed a lobulated mediastinal mass (*arrows*) the lower part of which was confused with an enlarged heart in this underexposed radiograph. **b** Lateral view chest radiograph showed that the lobulated mass was in a paraspinal location (*arrows*). **c** Film of the abdomen showing marked splenomegaly (*arrows*). *S*, spleen. **d** CT examination showing bilateral spinal masses (*M*) which represented extramedullary hematopoiesis. The fact that the mass was associated with splenomegally narrowed the differential diagnosis down to lymphoproliferative disorder such as lymphoma, leukemia, and extramedullary hematopoiesis

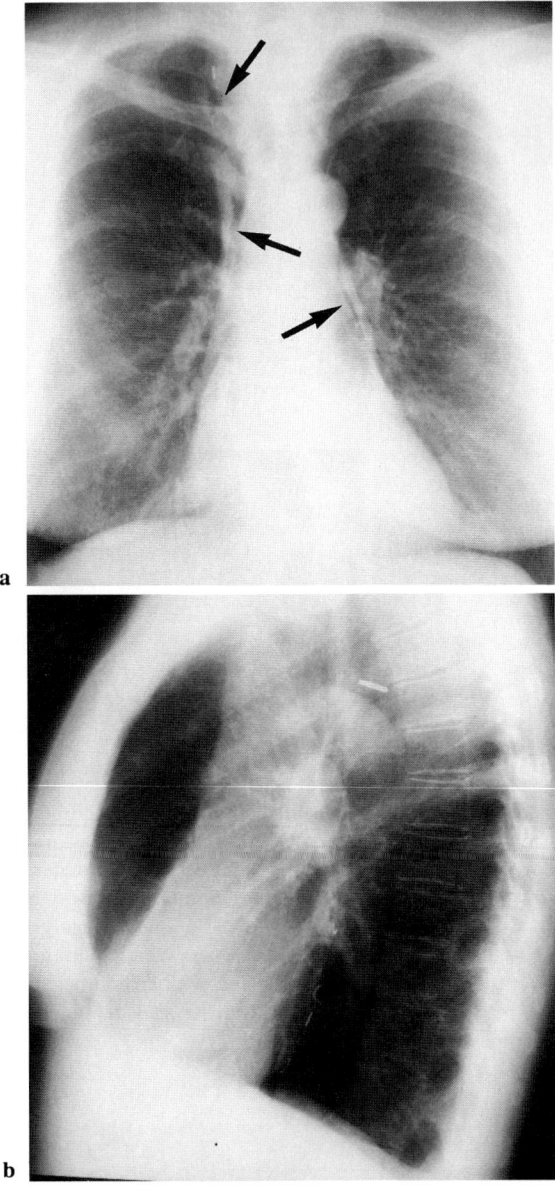

a

b

**Fig. 67a, b.** Importance of adequate knowledge of patient's clinical history. **a** Frontal view chest radiograph which I interpreted as showing pneumomediastinum (*arrows*). **b** Lateral view chest radiograph showed an air collection in the anterior mediastinum and a surgical clip. The X-ray referral did not include appropriate clinical history. When inquiring about the patient, the reason for the air in the mediastinum became quite apparent. The patient had had an esophageal carcinoma and had undergone surgical resection of the esophagus with gastric interposition. The air was in the relocated stomach

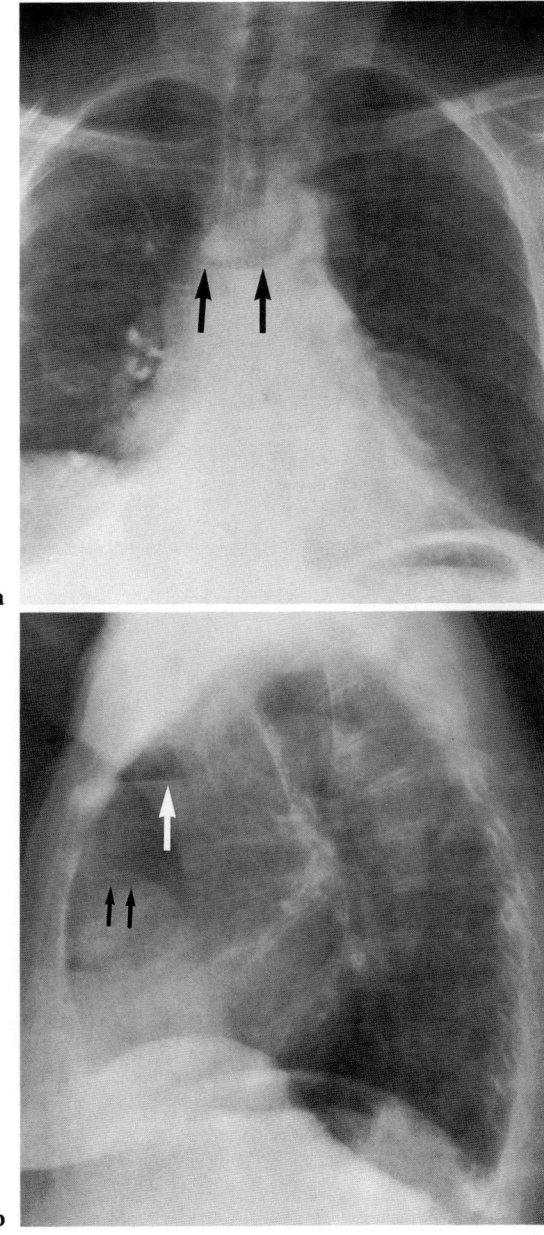

**Fig. 68a, b.** Importance of adequate knowledge of patient's clinical history. Colonic inter-position. **a** An air–fluid level was observed in the mediastinum (*arrows*). An abscess was considered. **b** A lateral view chest radiograph showed the air–fluid level in the anterior medi-astinum (*arrows*). The patient was asymptomatic, and on reviewing the history the diagnosis of colonic interposition was made based on the history of surgical resection of an esophageal carcinoma

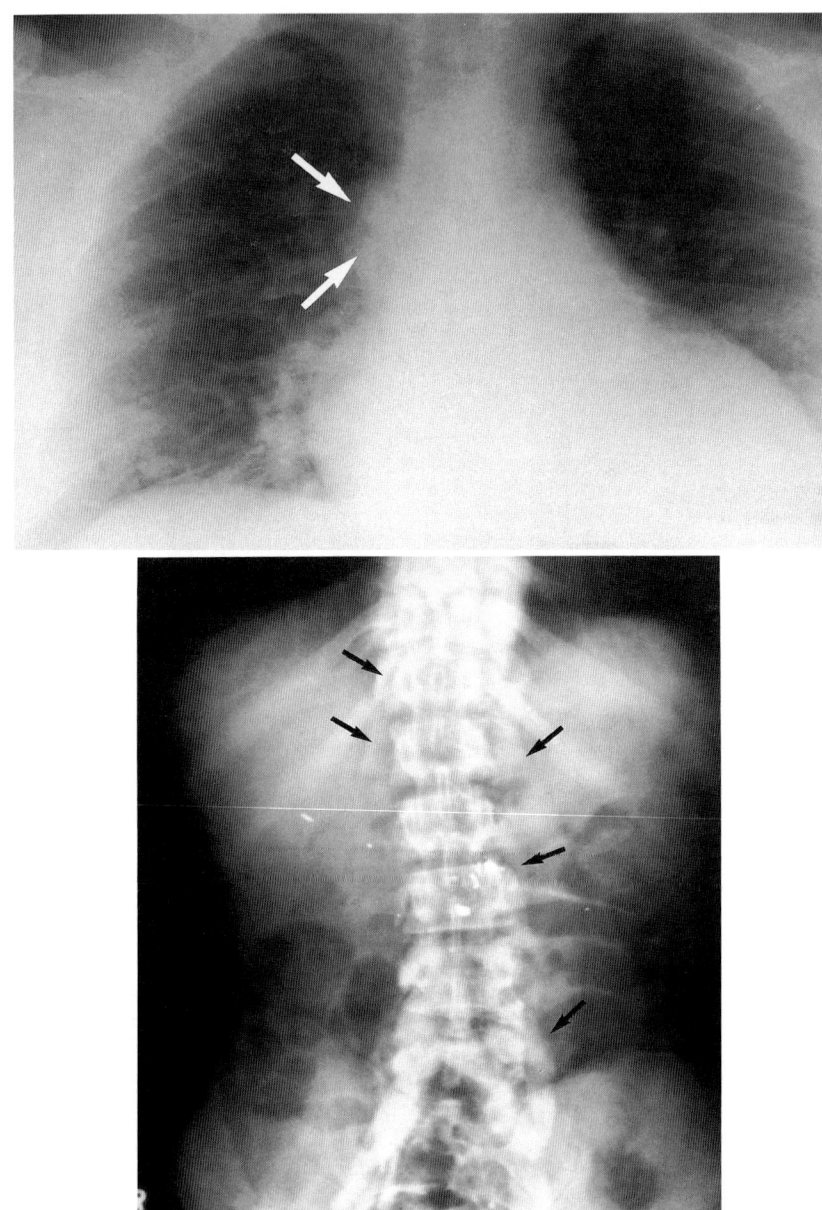

**Fig. 69a, b.** Importance of adequate knowledge of patient's clinical history. **a** A patient with a prominent azygos arch (*arrows*) and a history of leg edema should suggest a diagnosis of inferior vena cava obstruction. **b** Femoral vein injections of contrast media revealed total obstruction of the inferior vena cava and prominent collateral circulation (*arrows*). The patient was a drug addict and had injected his femoral veins which thrombosed and partially recanalized; the thrombus extended into the inferior vena cava

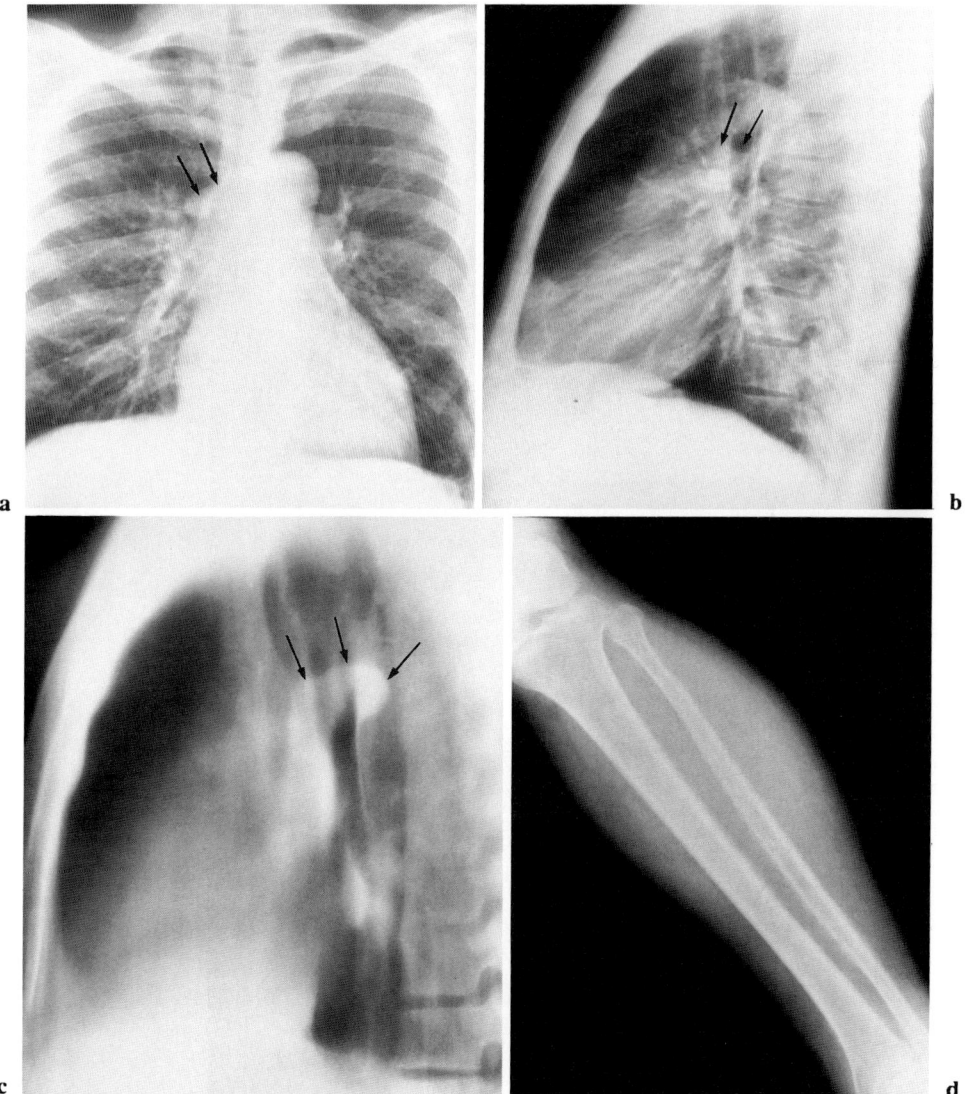

a

b

c

d

**Fig. 70a–d.** Importance of adequate knowledge of patient's clinical history. Drug addict with thrombosed inferior vena cava. **a** A prominent azygos arch (*arrows*) was observed in the frontal view chest radiograph. **b** A lateral view chest radiograph interpreted as normal. A prominent azygos arch was again noted (*arrows*). **c** Lateral view chest tomogram showing the enlarged azygos arch (*arrows*) as suspected in the lateral view chest radiograph. **d** Film of the leg showing edema. This was another drug addict with thrombosed inferior vena cava, the reason for collateral circulation to the azygos system

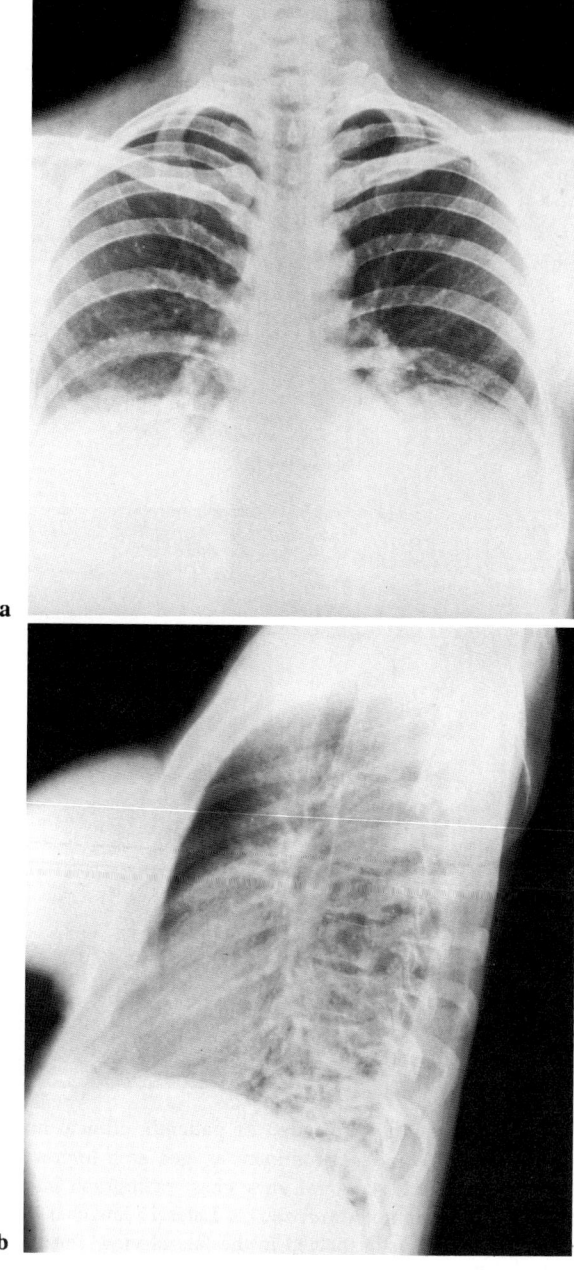

a

b

**Fig. 71a, b.** Importance of adequate knowledge of patient's clinical history. False subpulmonic effusion. **a** Frontal view chest radiograph in a female patient showed bilateral paracardiac masses. **b** A lateral view chest radiograph was ordered and revealed the presence of bilateral mammoplasty. The masses were not related to pulmonary, pleural, or diaphragmatic abnormalities. They were the result of mammoplasty

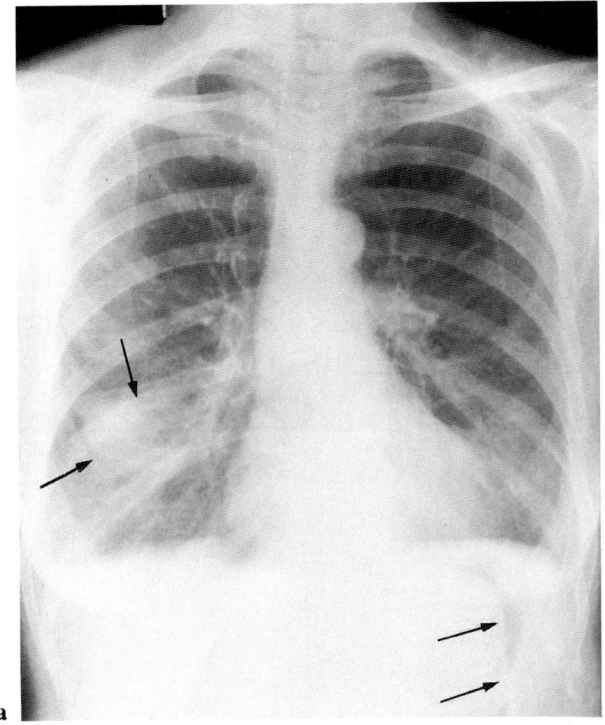

**Fig. 72a.** Importance of adequate knowledge of patient's clinical history. Bowen's disease. This patient had a bronchogenic carcinoma in the lower lobe of the right lung (*upper arrows*) and a suggestion of a mass in the stomach (*lower arrows*)

Bowen's disease is a specific variant of cutaneous intraepidermal squamous cell carcinoma (precancerous dermatosis; see Rickert et al. 1977). It occurs in both sexes and at all ages, but is most common in fair-complexioned white males, usually middle-aged or older. The lesion is more often solitary than multiple. It has a slow evolution. Approximately 6–7 years after the onset of Bowen's disease, 40% of patients will have developed additional premalignant and malignant cutaneous and mucocutaneous lesions. More than 10% will have multiple combinations.

Extracutaneous cancers that have been described in Bowen's disease include those of the respiratory, gastrointestinal, genitourinary, and reticuloendothelial systems, as well as of the oral cavity, breast, endocrine system, soft tissues, and mucous membranes of the lip, eye, and anus. Incidence is higher when Bowen's disease has occurred on nonsolar-exposed skin. Five percent occur at multiple anatomic sites and 5% have occult cancers.

The patient should be under continuous clinical surveillance because of the possibillity that another, more serious neoplasm may either coexist or subsequently develop.

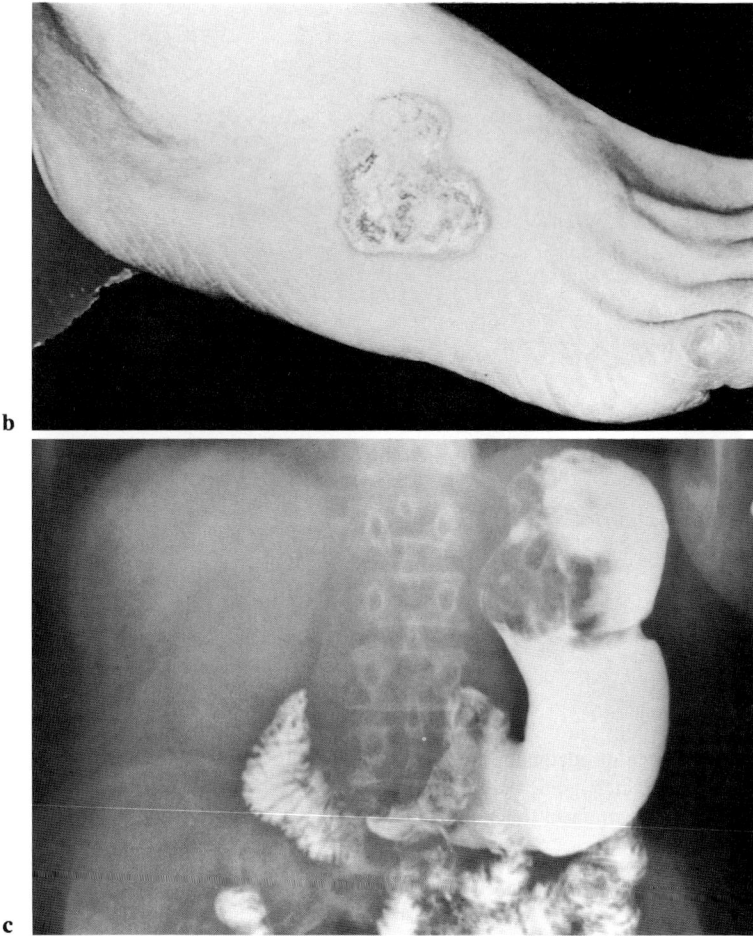

b

c

**Fig. 72b, c.** Importance of adequate knowledge of patient's clinical history. Bowen's disease.
**b** The patient presented with a chronic skin ulcer. **c** An upper GI series revealed a carcinoma
of the stomach. Synchronous carcinomas were present

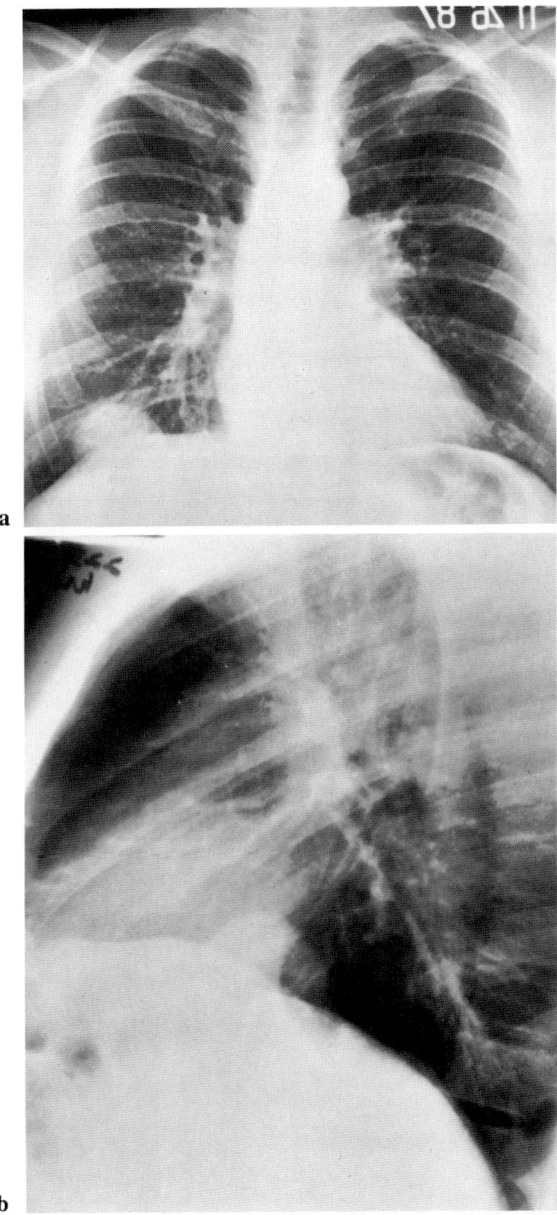

a

b

**Fig. 73a, b.** Importance of adequate knowledge of patient's clinical history. The patient had trauma to the right upper quadrant. A nodule was shown adjacent to the right hemidiaphragm in both frontal (**a**) and lateral (**b**) views of the chest. Because of the history of trauma, a liver scan revealed that the uptake of this nodule was identical to the liver. This is an example of intrathoracic liver secondary to diaphragmatic rupture and migration of the liver tissue into the chest

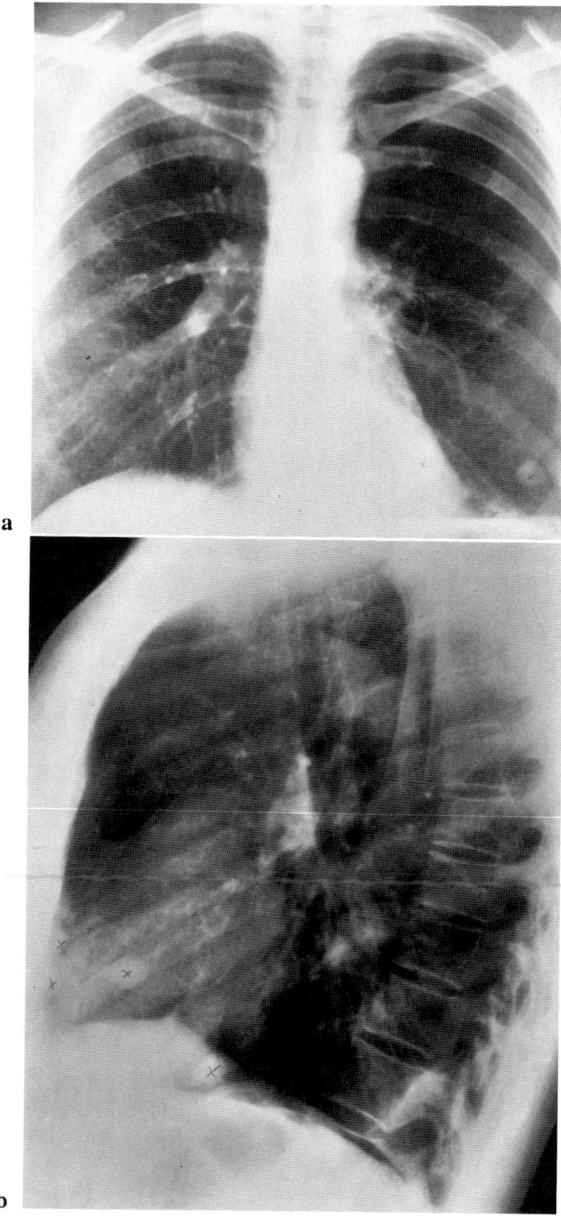

a

b

**Fig. 74a, b.** Importance of adequate knowledge of patient's clinical history. The patient had trauma to the left upper quadrant. Several nodules appeared on the periphery of the left hemithorax (nodules are marked with an *X*). There is seen in both the frontal (a) and lateral (b) views of the chest. A splenic scan showed the uptake of these nodules to suggest intrathoracic splenosis. In the differential diagnosis of solitary or multiple nodules in the left hemithorax, a history of trauma should be considered. These nodules represent migration and growth of splenic tissue in the left hemithorax. They are usually peripherally located and may be multiple: they are mostly found adjacent to the diaphragm

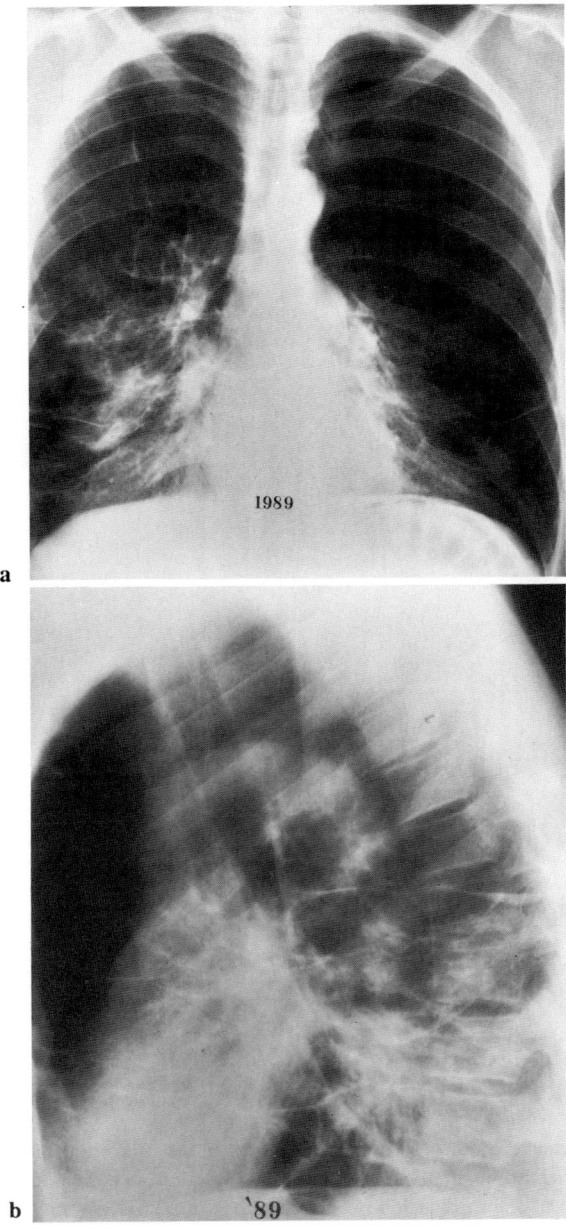

**Fig. 75a, b.** Importance of adequate knowledge of patient's clinical history. The patient was known to have AIDS. Frontal (**a**) and lateral (**b**) views of the chest revealed bullous changes affecting both upper lobes. The patient had no history of smoking nor evidence of $\alpha_1$-antitrypsin globulin deficiency. In the latter, the bullous changes are usually present in the lower zones. Here the changes were present primarily in the upper lobes. This is an example of AIDS-related pulmonary cysts. Knowledge of the patient's history of AIDS was useful in diagnosing the etiology of the pulmonary changes

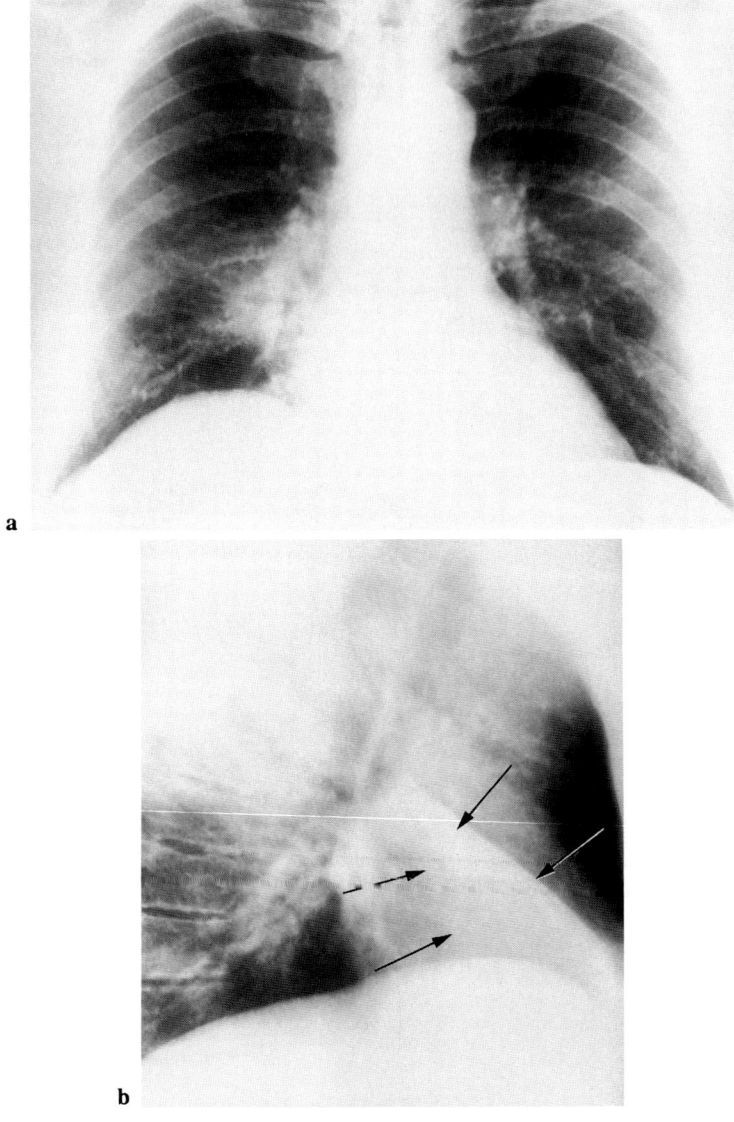

a

b

**Fig. 76a, b.** Importance of careful examination of the hila. **a** Frontal view chest radiograph interpreted as a pneumonia in the right perihilar region. **b** Lateral view chest radiograph showing atelectasis of the middle lobe secondary to a proximal obstructing bronchial carcinoma

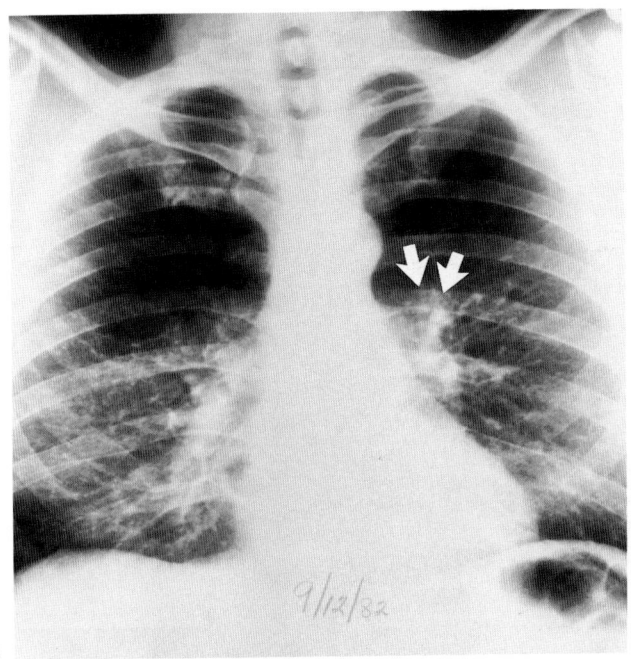

a

**Fig. 77a.** Importance of careful examination of the hila. Missed bronchial carcinoma. Ill-defined density around left hilum was noted on 12 September 1982 (*arrows*). The patient was asymptomatic

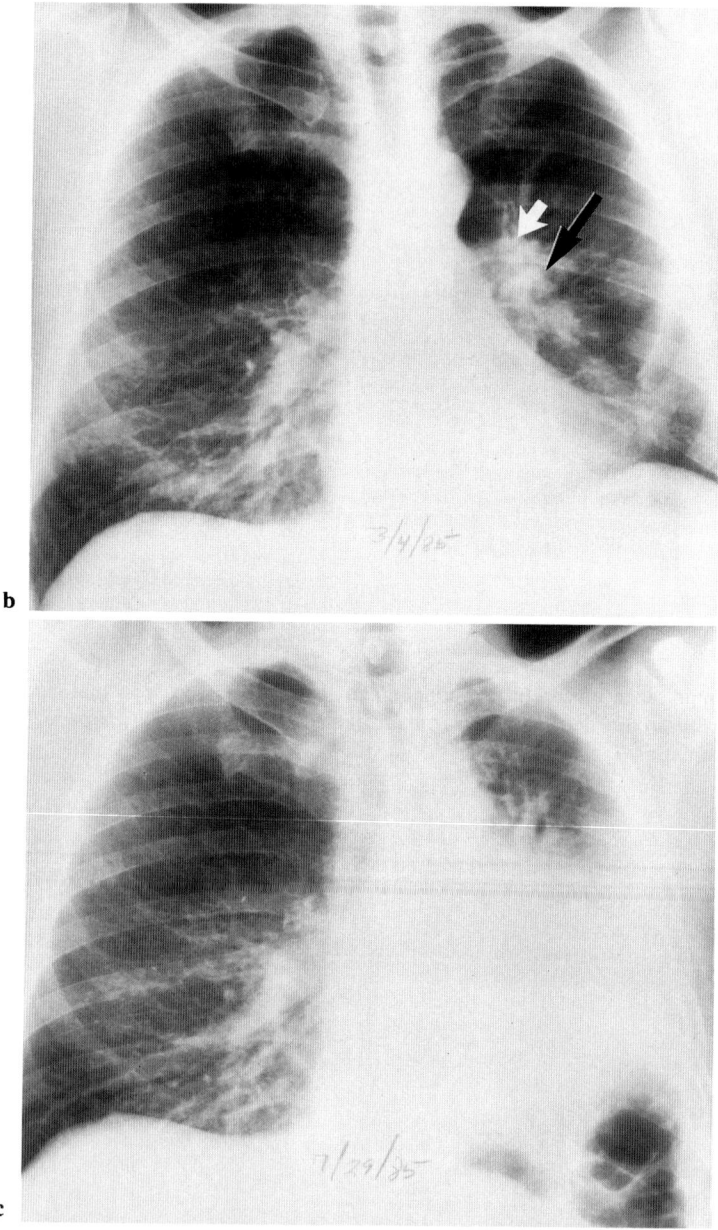

**Fig. 77b, c.** Importance of careful examination of the hila. Missed bronchial carcinoma. **b** On 4 March 1985, the perihilar mass had become enlarged and proved to be a bronchial carcinoma (*arrows*). The carcinoma was already present in 1982 and was overlooked in this patient with chronic obstructive pulmonary disease. **c** By 29 July 1985, unilateral lymphangitic spread had occurred

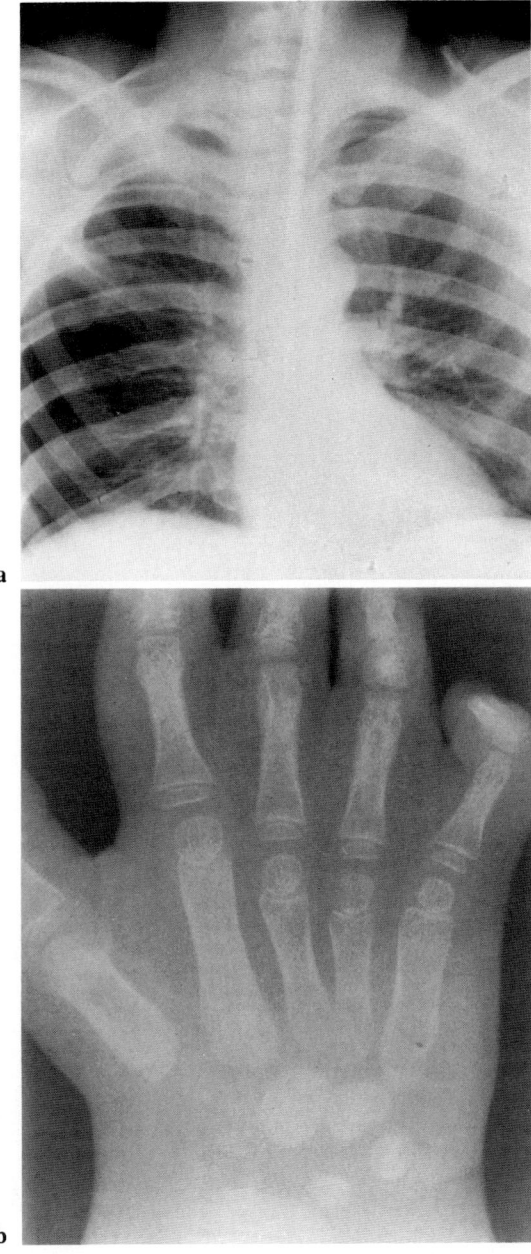

a

b

**Fig. 78a, b.** Learn about your patient. **a** Patient with hyperlucency involving the lower half of the right lung. The patient also had ipsilateral syndactylism of the fingers of his right hand. **b** Film of the right hand of a patient with the same process (Poland syndrome). This is the result of agenesis of the pectoralis major which can simulate an area of parenchymal disease or vascular insufficiency

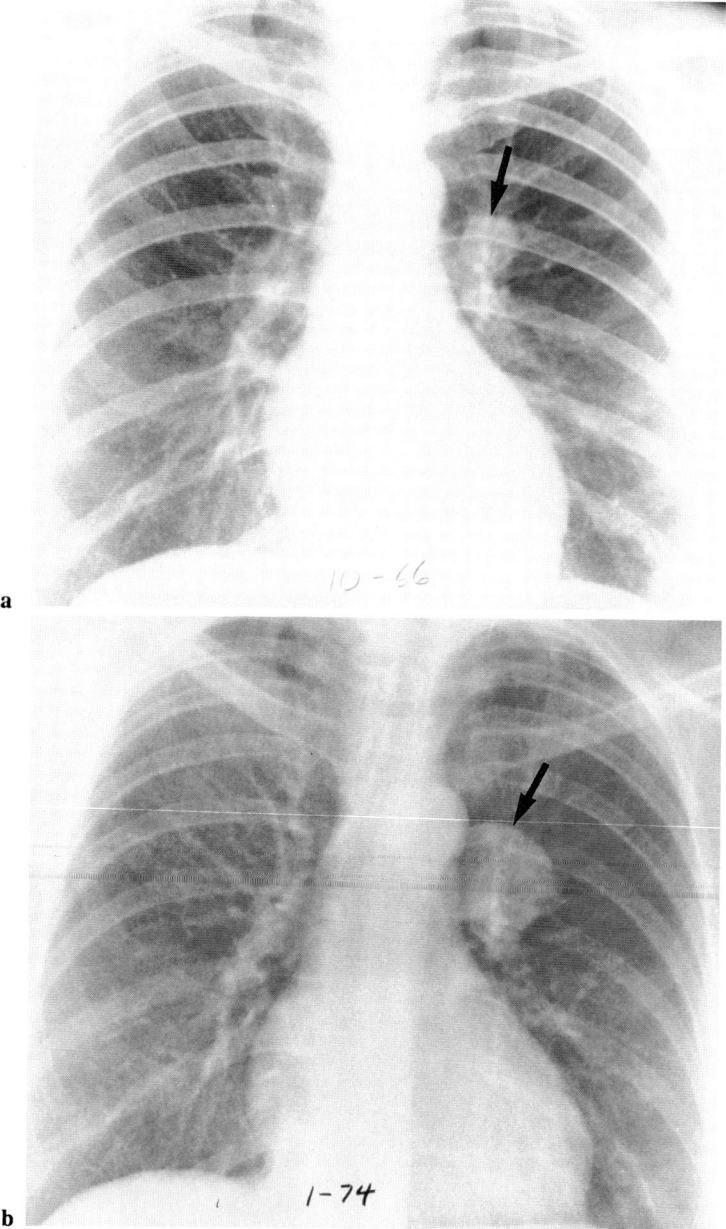

**Fig. 79a, b.** Don't procrastinate. **a** Nodule in the left juxtahilar region (*arrow*). In this 28-year-old asymptomatic woman, the nodule was believed to represent a benign condition. She was a nonsmoker. **b** Films taken 8 years later showed the growth of that mass (*arrow*). There was no interval chest radiographic examination. The lesion was resected and proved to be a bronchial carcinoid

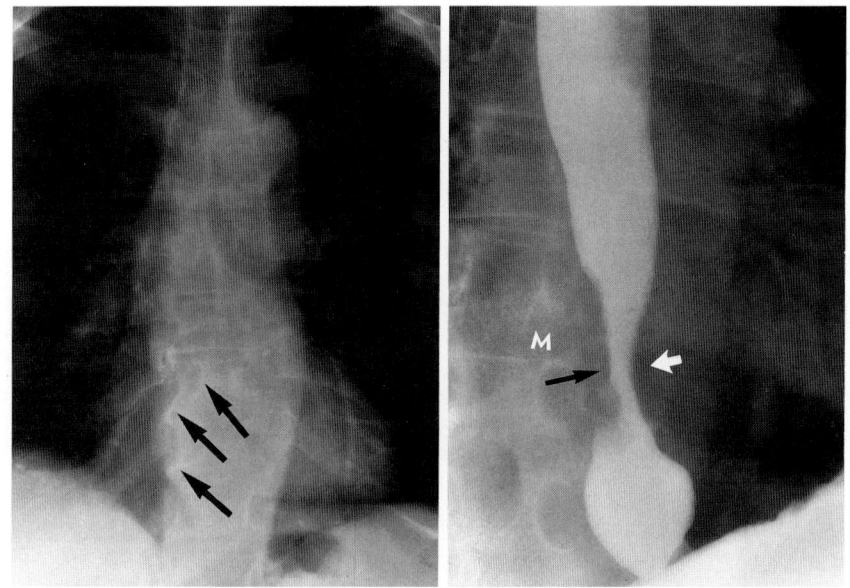

a                                                                    b

**Fig. 80a, b.** The value of the esophagogram. 68-year-old man with progressive dysphagia, first to solids and then to liquids, and who had lost 30 lb over a short period of time. **a** Penetrated frontal view of the chest shows displaced pleuroazygoesophageal line in its lower third (*arrows*). **b** Barium swallow revealed smooth narrowing of the distal esophagus (*arrows*) and a paraesophageal mass (*M*). With the history and these findings, the plain radiograph suggested the correct diagnosis of an esophageal carcinoma

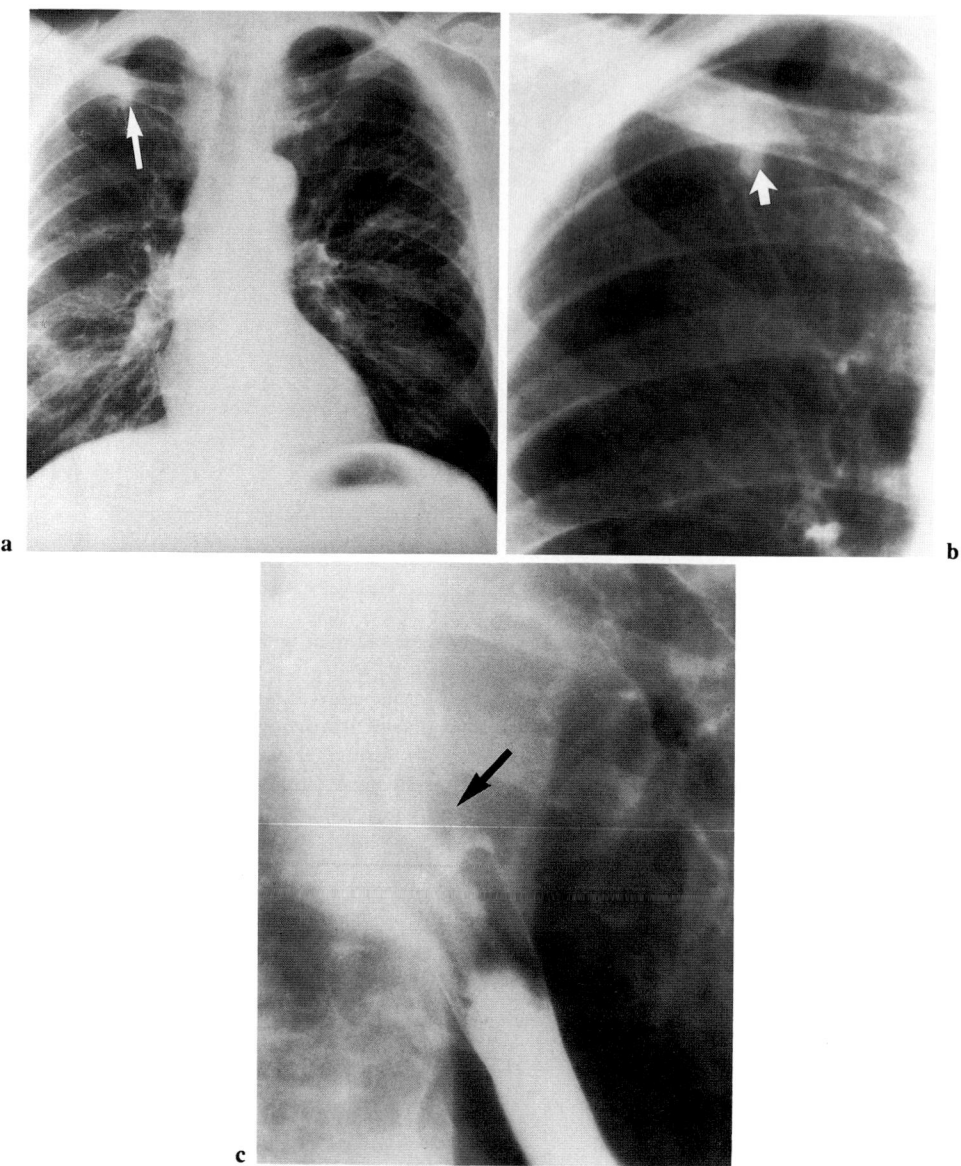

a

b

c

Fig. 81a–c. Value of an esophagogram. Patient with dysphagia. **a, b** Plain chest roentgeno-gram revealed an irregular nodule in the upper lobe of the right lung (*arrows*). **c** Barium swallow where a lesion could be observed in the mid-thoracic esophagus (*arrow*). This proved to be a bronchogenic carcinoma with metastasis to the esophagus

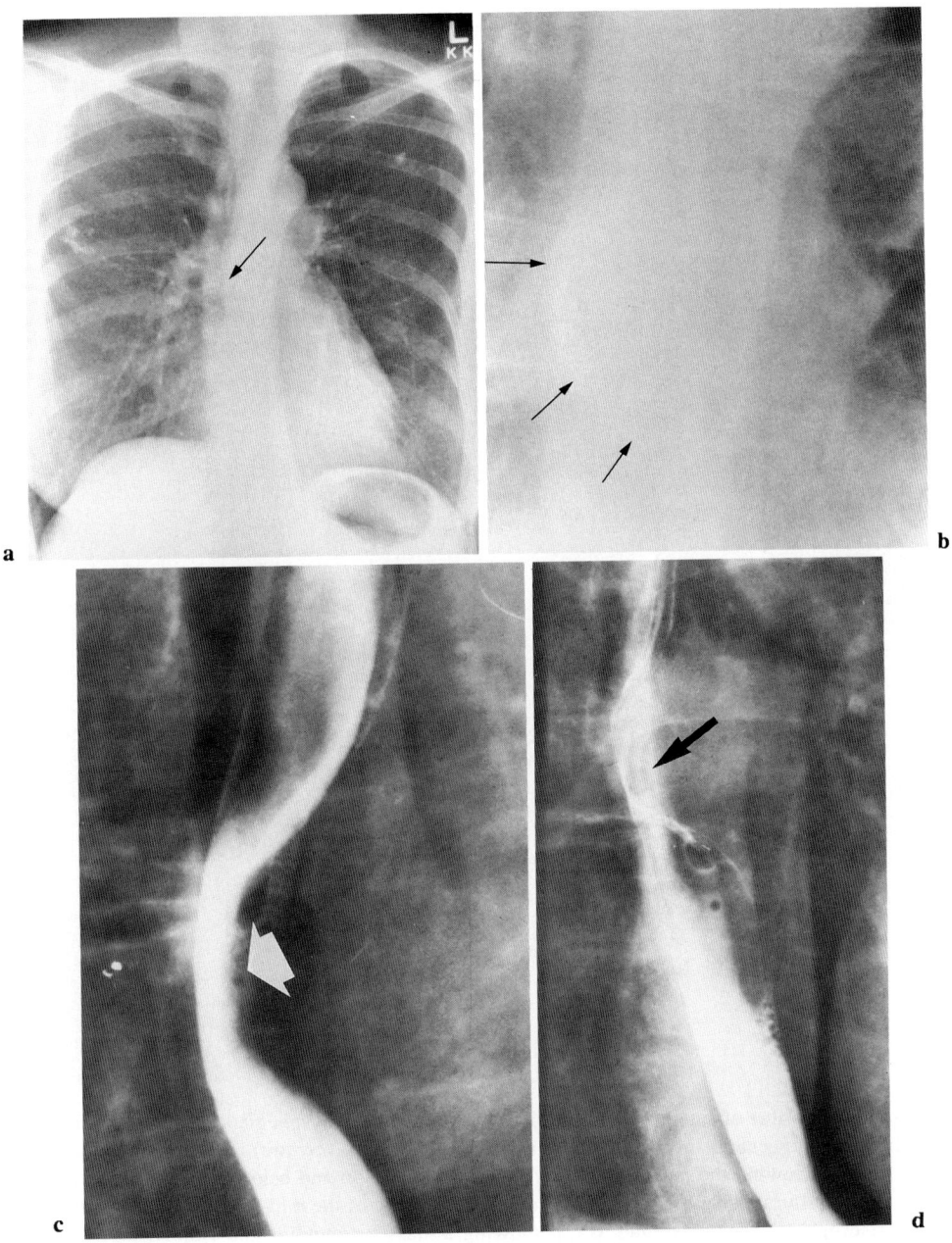

**Fig. 82a–d.** Value of an esophagogram. Patient with dysphagia and a fibrocalcific lesion in the right mid-lung field. **a** In the frontal view, a displaced pleuroazygoesophageal line (*arrow*) was noted. **b** Close-up suggesting the presence of a subcarinal mass displacing the pleuroazygoesophageal line (*arrows*). **c, d** Barium swallowing showed smooth eccentric esophageal mass (*arrows*) which proved to be metastatic bronchogenic carcinoma

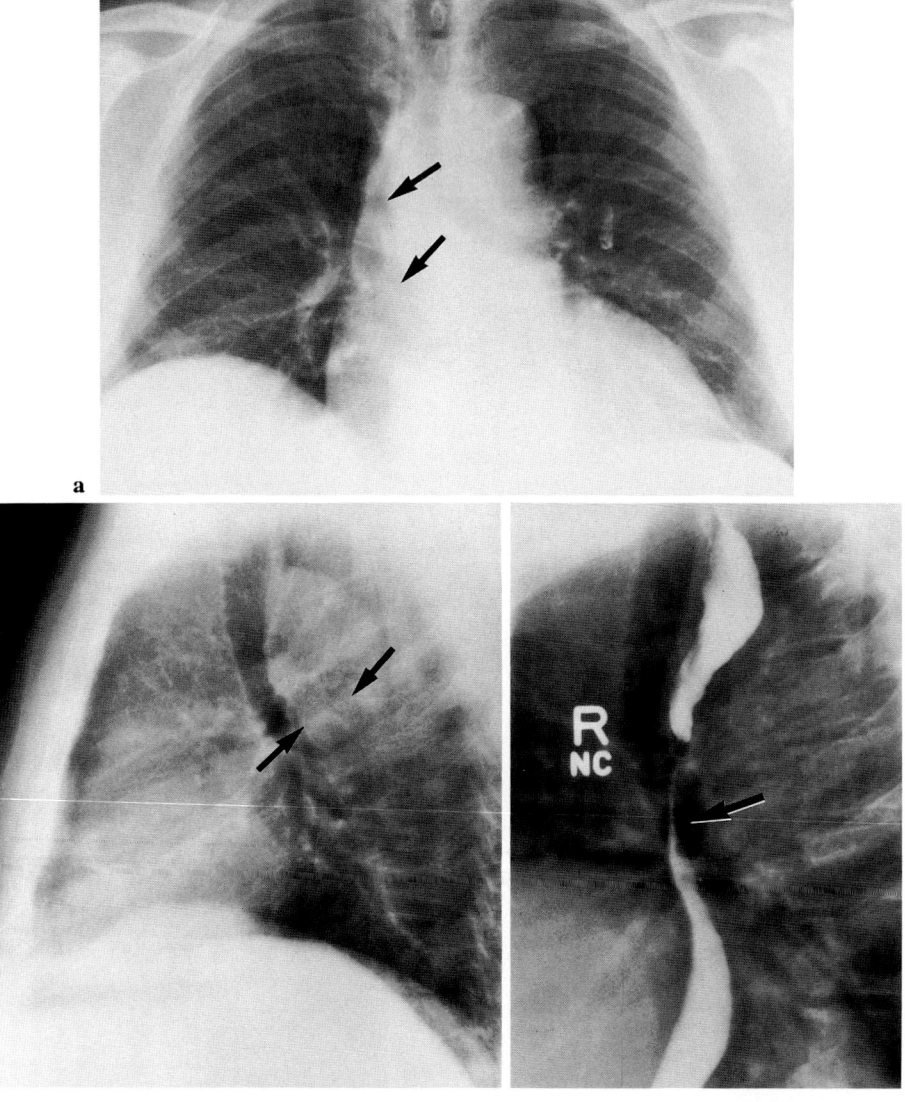

a

b                                                                                    c

**Fig. 83a–e.** Value of esophagogram. Elderly individual with dysphagia. **a** Frontal view chest radiograph suggesting the presence of a retrocardiac mass (*arrows*). **b** Lateral view chest radiograph showing the mass behind the tracheal bifurcation and below the arch of the aorta (*arrows*). **c** Barium swallow revealed a smooth narrowing of the mid-thoracic esophagus with a juxtaesophageal mass (*arrow*). **d** CT showing a mass surrounding the esophagus. **e** CT of the upper abdomen showing paraaortic nodes (*arrow*). The patient had a primary esophageal cancer with extensive metastasis to the periesophageal and periaortic nodes

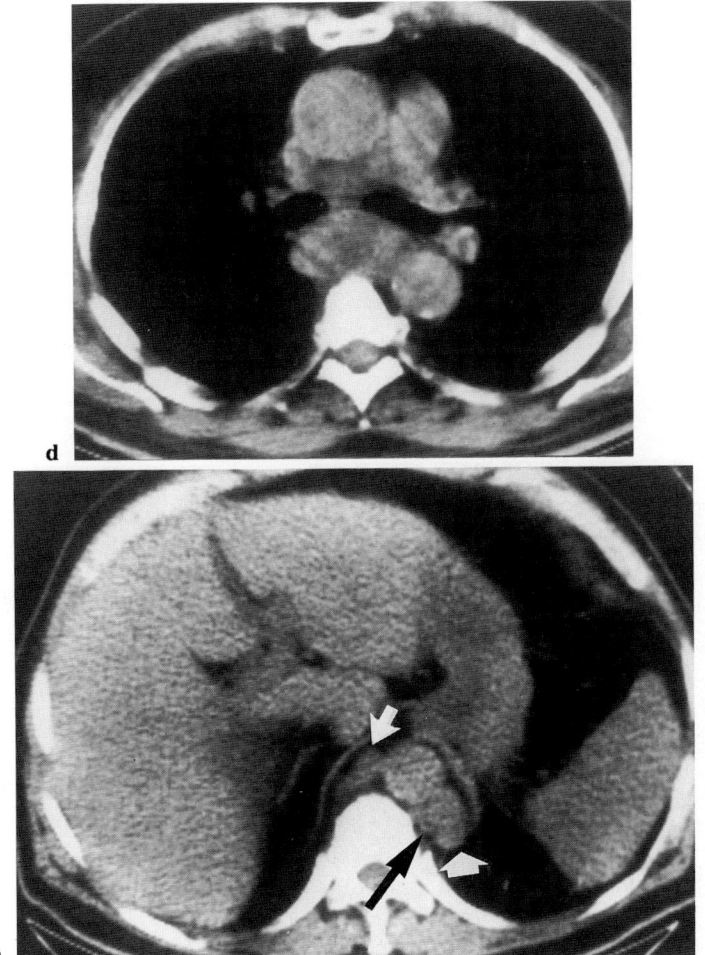

d

e

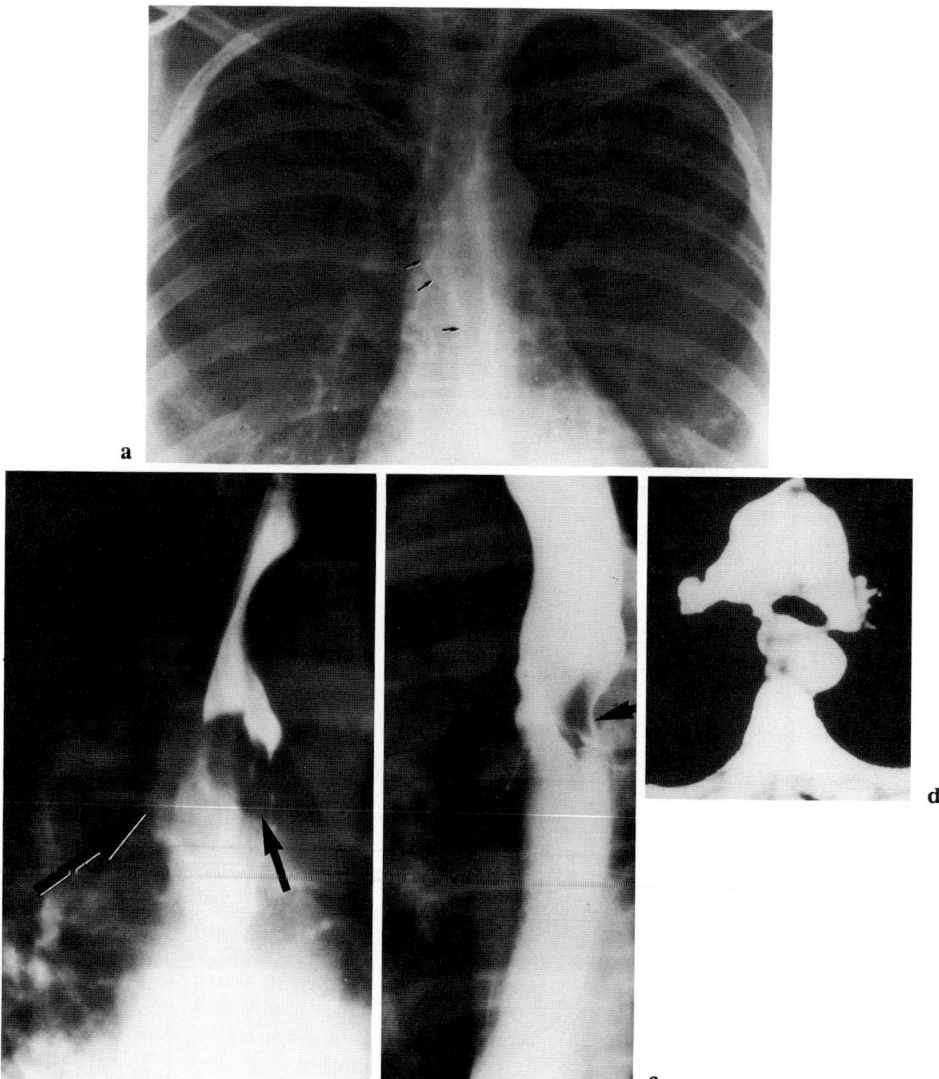

**Fig. 84a–d.** Value of esophagogram. Primary esophageal cancer. **a** Frontal view chest radiograph. Note displacement of the pleuroazygoesophageal line (*arrows*). **b, c** Barium swallows showing esophageal lesion (*arrows*). **d** CT. The perioesophageal mass represented a carcinoma of the esophagus

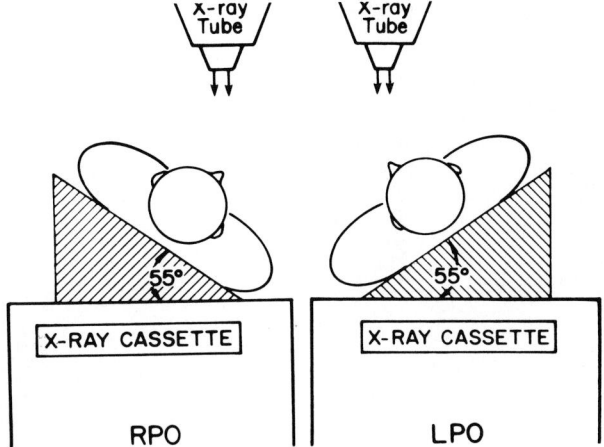

**Fig. 85.** Oblique tomography angles for the hila. Note that conventional wedges are 45°, whereas these are 55°

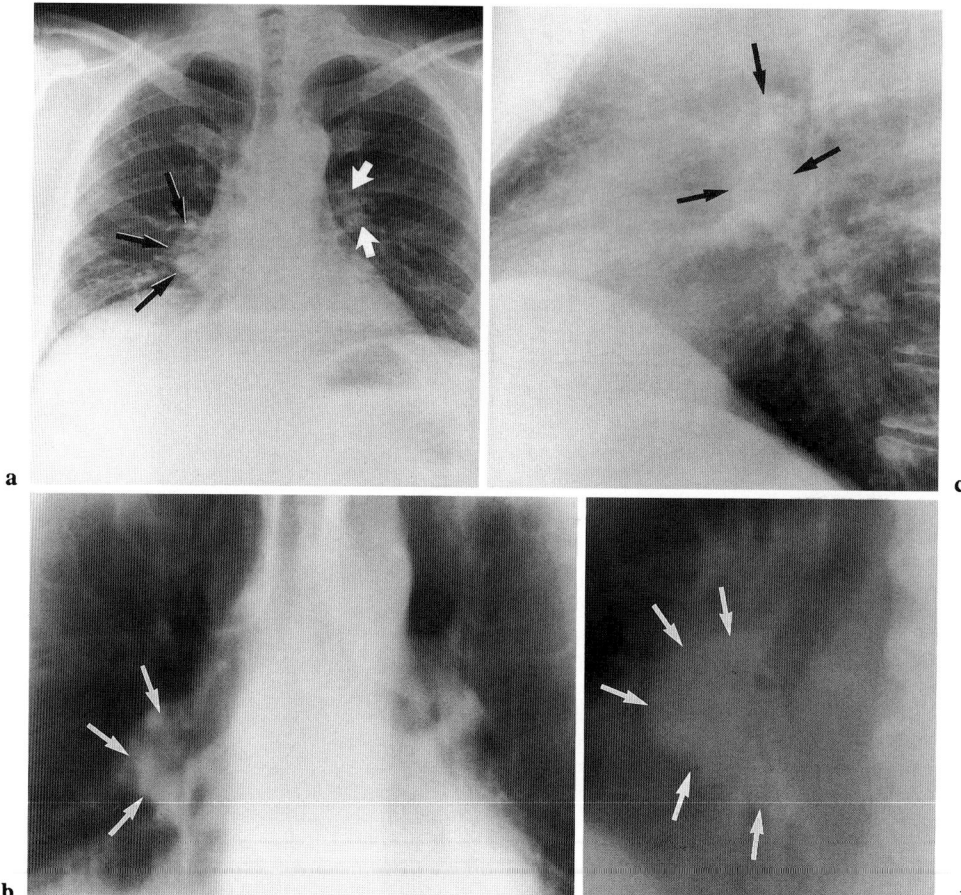

**Fig. 86a–d.** Value of linear tomography of the hilum. Patient with a history of melanoma. **a** Frontal view chest radiograph showed poor inspiratory effort and prominence of the hilar shadows (*arrows*). **b** Lateral view chest radiograph of the same patient showing prominence of the hilar shadows (*arrows*). **c** Frontal and **d** right posterior oblique tomographs revealing lobulated mass in right hilar region (*arrows*) that proved to be metastatic melanoma. Linear tomography clarified the nonvascular nature of the mediastinal mass

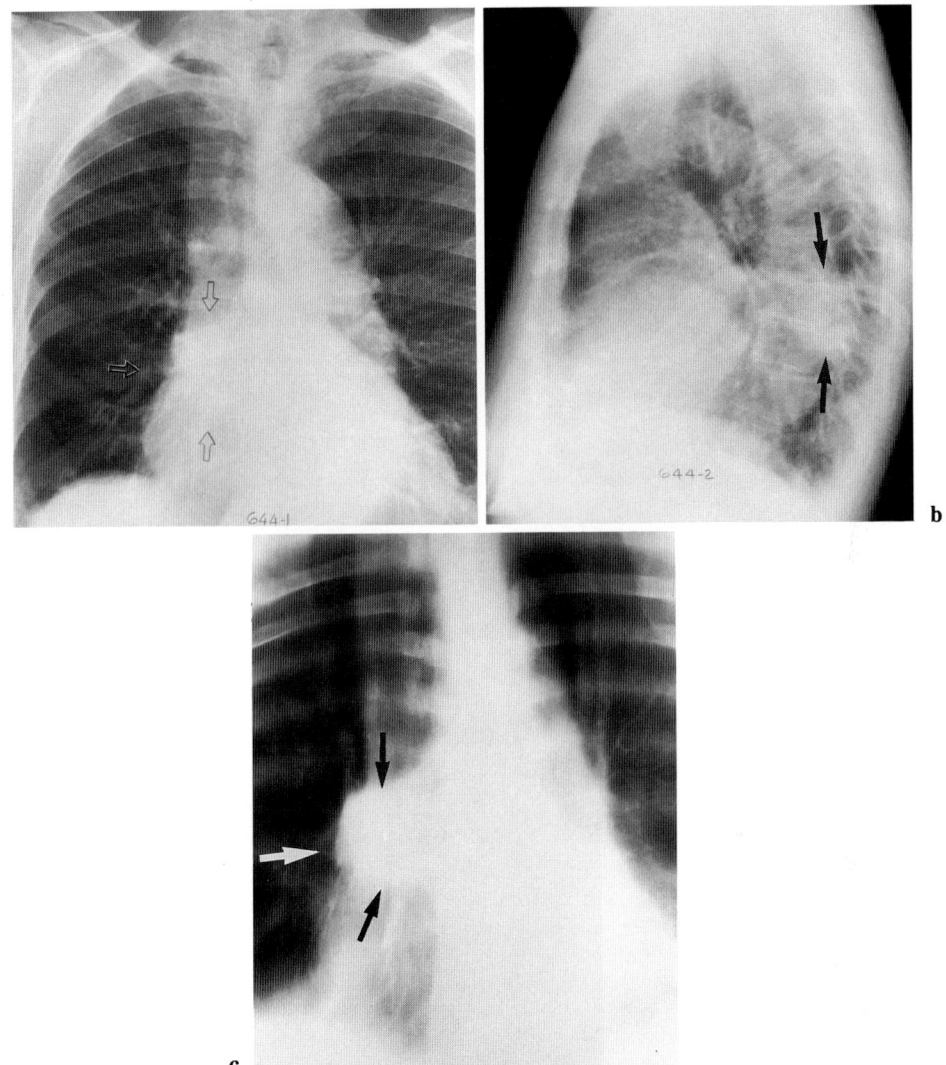

**Fig. 87a–c.** Value of linear tomography. **a** Frontal view chest radiograph showing an ill-defined mass in the retrocardiac region (*arrows*). **b** Lateral view chest radiograph showing a mass projected in the right paraspinal region (*arrows*). **c** Linear tomography revealing a mass with irregular outline (*arrows*). A bronchogenic carcinoma was suspected and confirmed at surgery

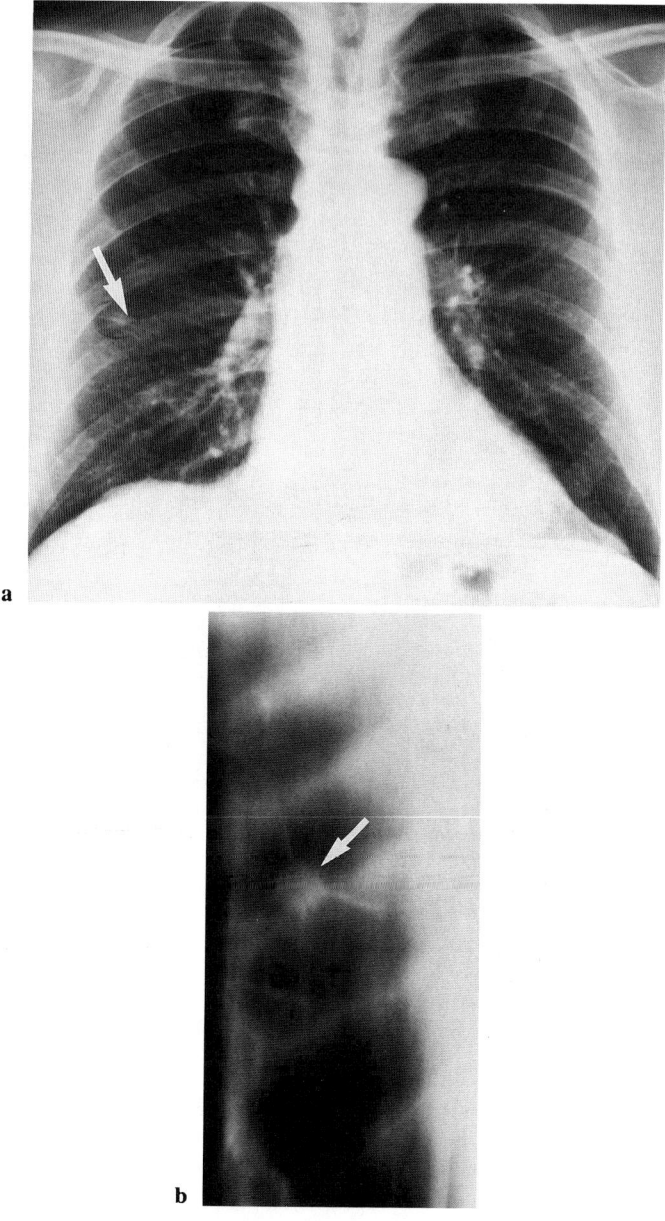

a

b

**Fig. 88a, b.** Value of linear tomography. **a** Frontal view chest radiograph showing an ill-defined nodule in the right mid-lung field (*arrow*). **b** Tomogram confirmed a nodule with spiculated margins (*arrow*). It proved to represent a peripheral adenocarcinoma

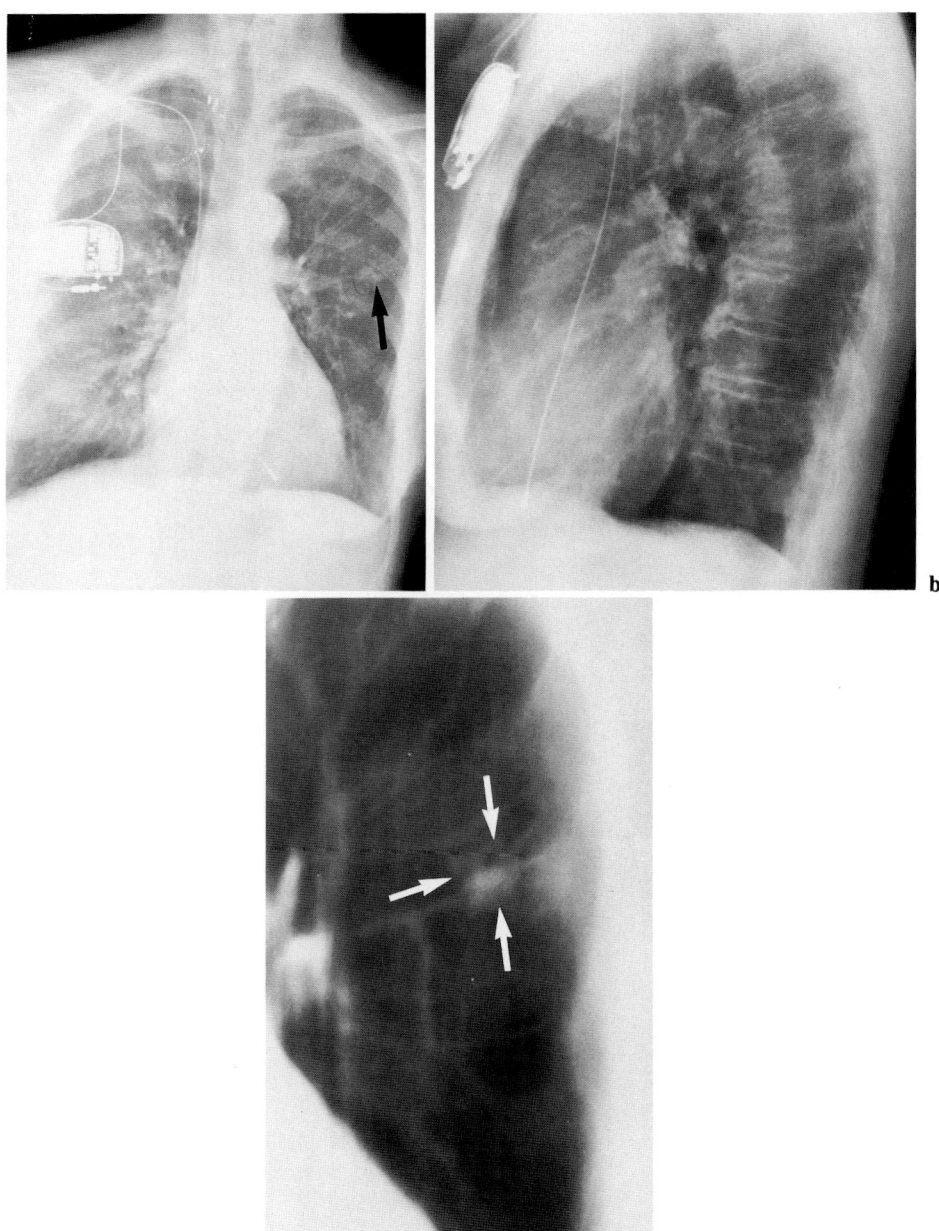

**Fig. 89a–c.** Value of linear tomography. **a** Frontal view chest radiograph showing ill-defined irregularity in the left mid-lung field *(arrow)*. **b** Lateral view chest radiograph failed to demonstrate the exact anatomic location of the abnormality. **c** Linear tomography confirmed the presence of an irregular, small nodule which proved to be a bronchial carcinoma *(arrows)*

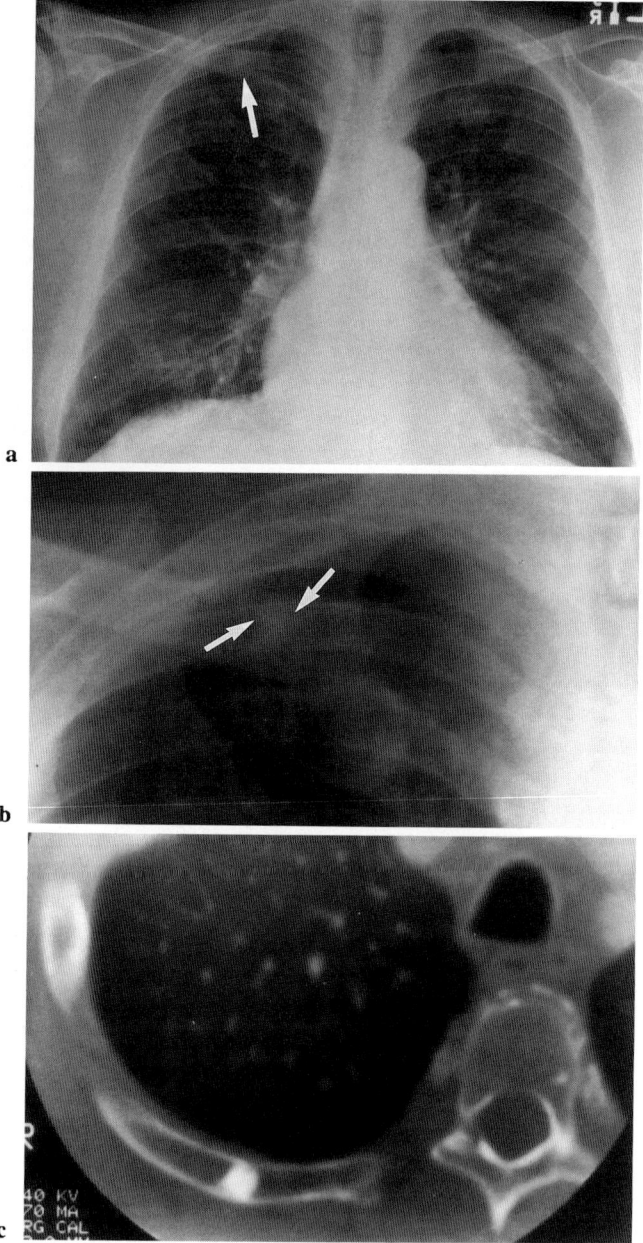

**Fig. 90a–c.** Value of CT for assessing the nature and stage of pulmonary nodules. Osteoma.
**a** Ill-defined nodular density in the right apex (*arrow*). **b** Close-up of the right apex showing
the ill-defined nodule (*arrows*). **c** CT of the right apex showing that the lesion was not in
the lung but in a rib and represented an osteoma

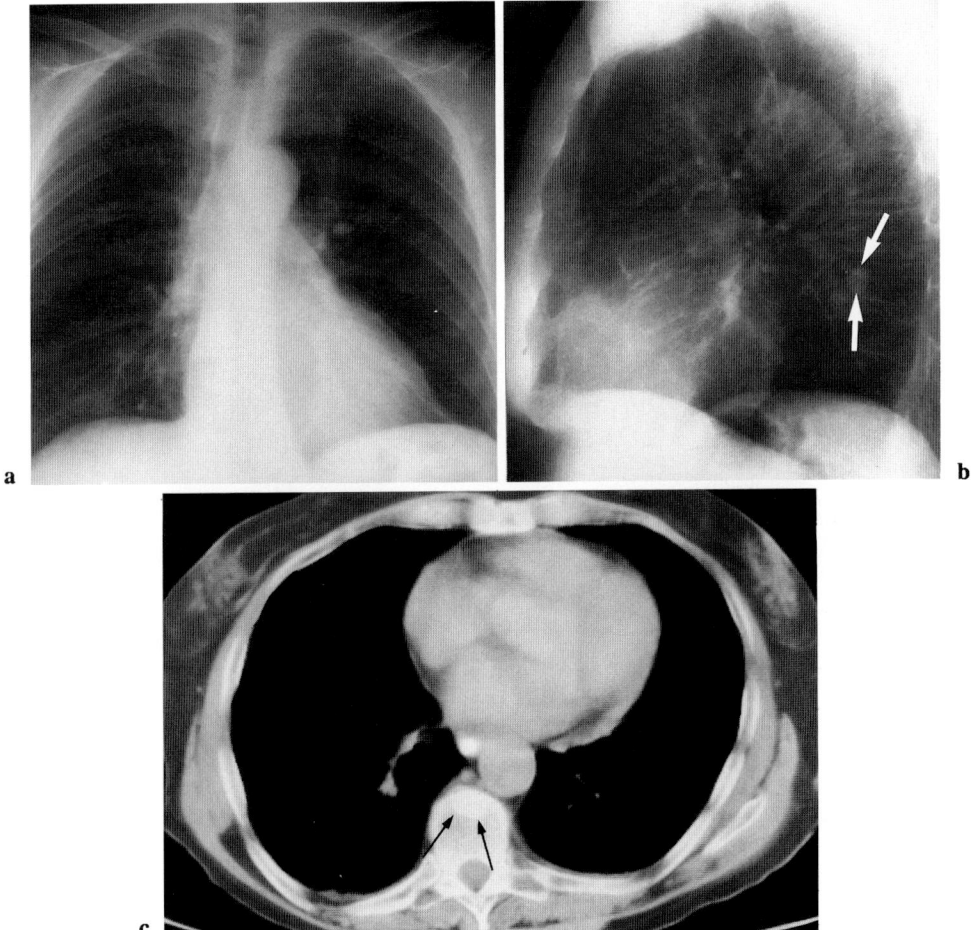

**Fig. 91a–c.** Value of CT for assessing the nature and stage of pulmonary nodules. Osteoma of the vertebral body. **a** Penetrated chest radiograph showing no abnormality whatsoever. **b** In the lateral view chest radiograph, an ill-defined nodular density was noted superimposed in the projection of the mid-thoracic spine (*arrows*). **c** CT showed that the lesion represented an osteoma of the vertebral body (*arrows*)

124

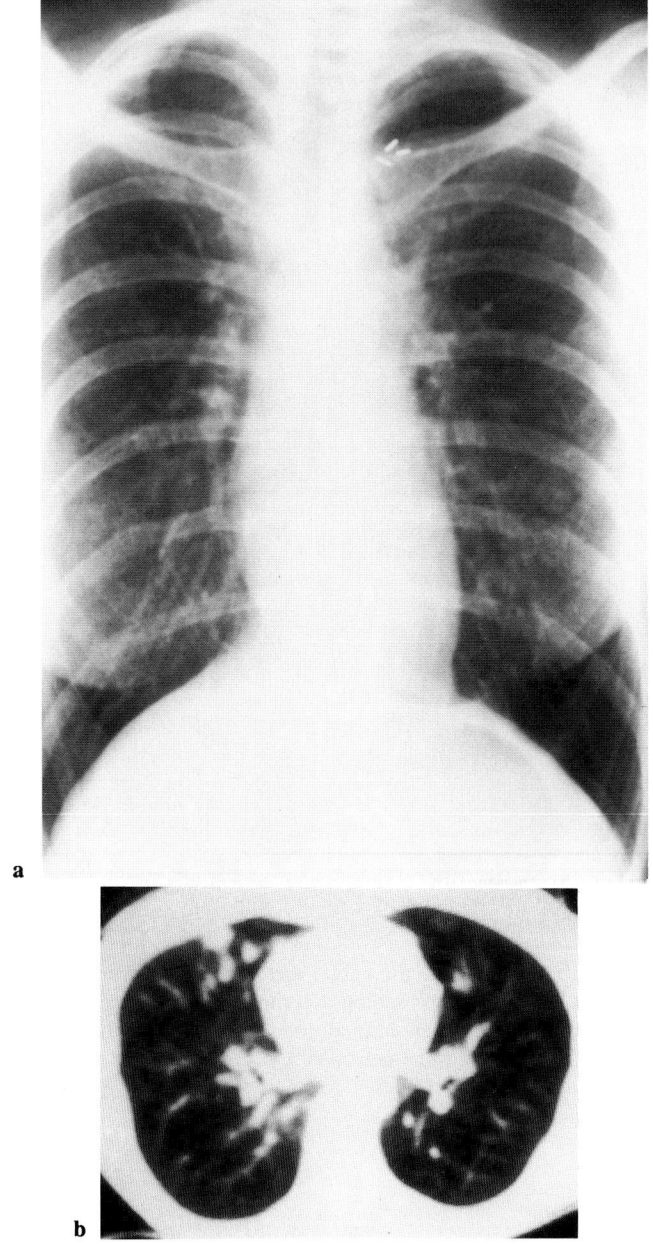

**Fig. 92a, b.** Value of CT for assessing pulmonary nodules. **a** Frontal view chest radiograph of woman with a rhabdomyosarcoma. Surgical slips were seen in the upper mediastinum. **b** CT showed multiple pulmonary nodules which represented metastatic disease, not seen on frontal view chest radiographs

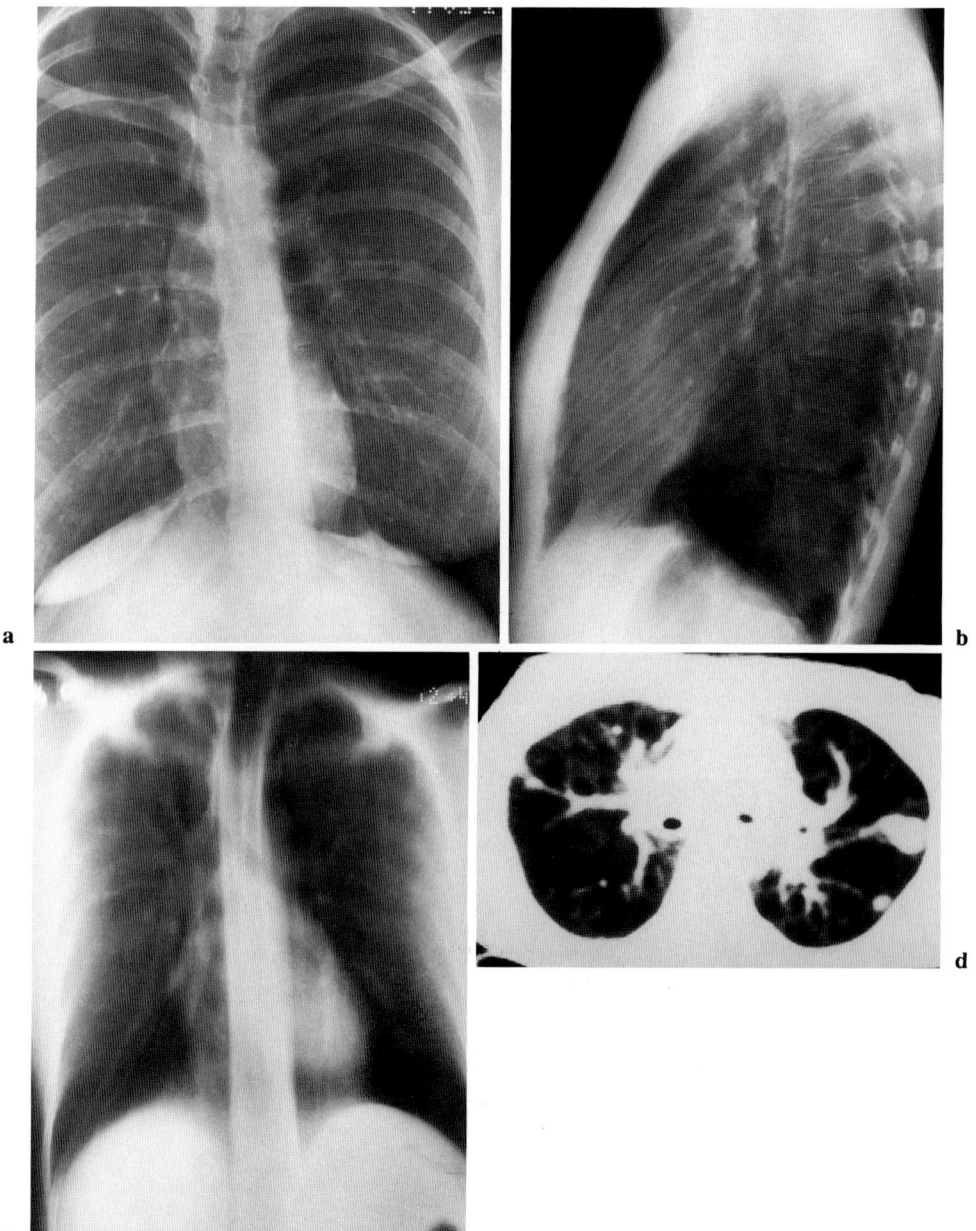

**Fig. 93a–d.** Value of CT for assessing pulmonary nodules. **a** Frontal and **b** lateral view chest radiographs showing no abnormalities. **c** Full chest linear tomography failed to demonstrate nodular densities. **d** CT of the chest revealing multiple pulmonary nodules, some quite large that proved to be metastatic disease

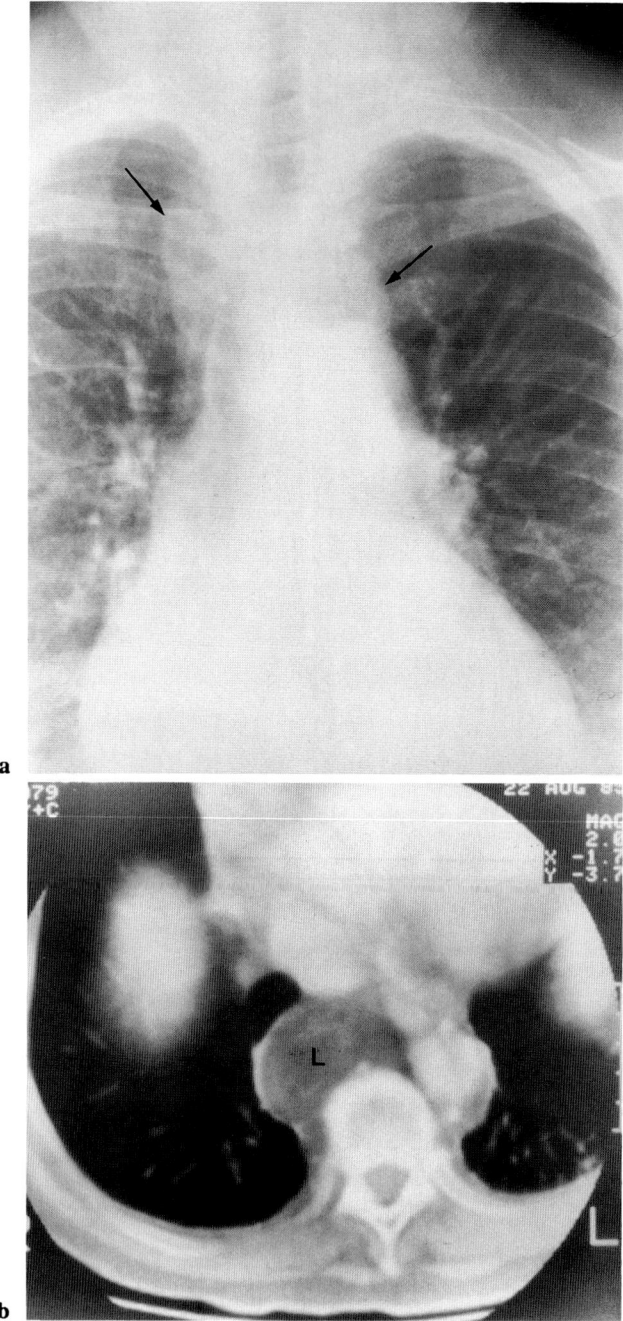

**Fig. 94a, b.** Value of CT for assessing pulmonary nodules. **a** Widened superior mediastinum (*arrows*) and apparent enlargement of the heart. **b** CT of the lower chest showing a fatty mass which extended along the right paravertebral region and with typical features of a lipoma

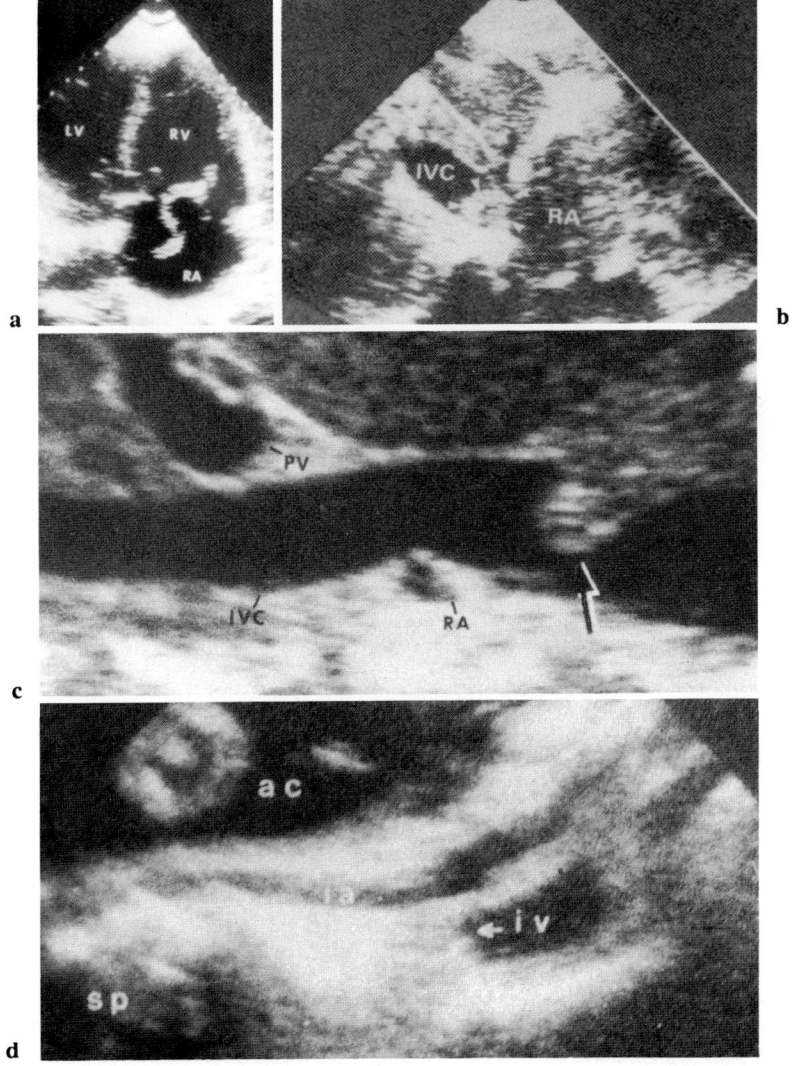

**Fig. 95a–d.** Value of ultrasonography in the workup of a radiolucency. **a** Sonogram showing mass in the right atrium (*RA*) projecting into the cavity of the right ventricle (*RV*), features that suggested a thrombus. This was the site of embolization of the lung. *LV*, left ventricle. **b** Thrombus (*arrows*) in the lumen of the inferior vena cava (*IVC*). *RA*, right atrium. **C** Thrombus in the inferior vena cava (*arrow*). *PV*, portal vein; *RA*, renal artery; *IVC*, inferior vena cava. **d** Occlusion of iliac vein (*IV*) due to a thrombus (*arrow*). *SP*, spine: *AC*, amniotic cavity; *IA*, iliac artery

128

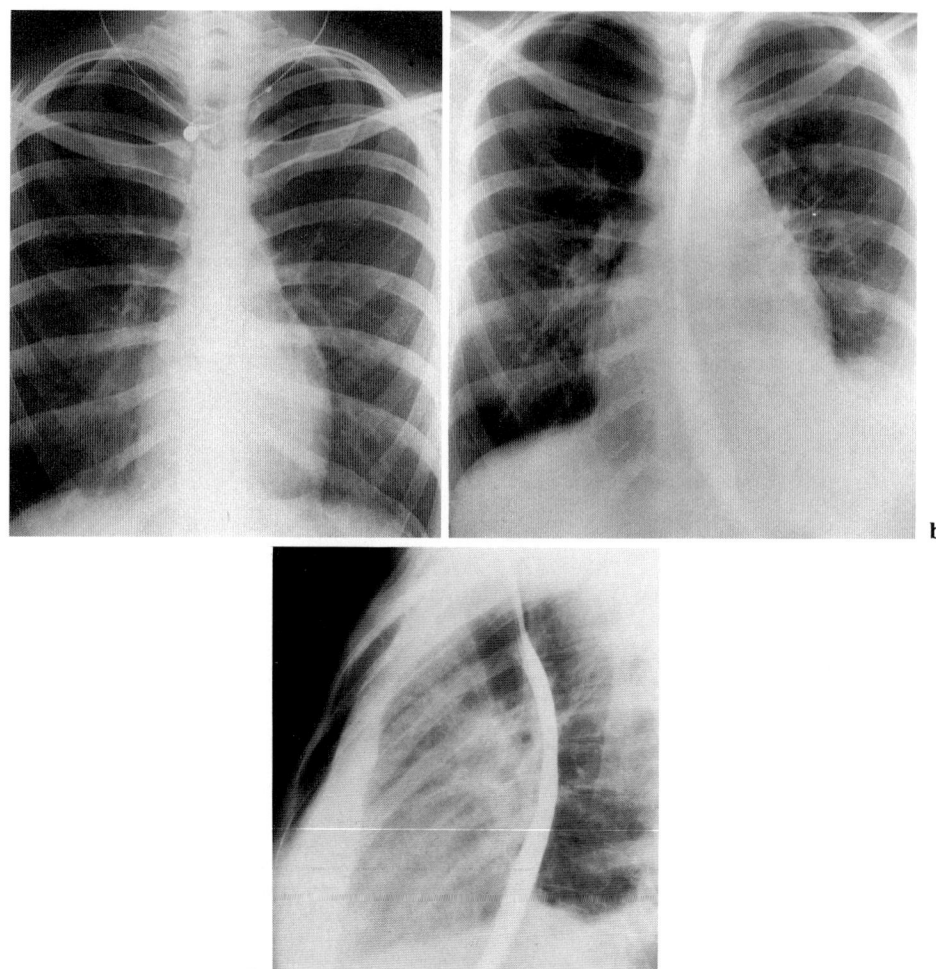

a

b

c

**Fig. 96a–c.** Value of arteriogram. Malignant mesenchymoma of the anterior mediastinum. 18-year-old woman who had a negative chest radiograph (**a**) a year before she developed acute chest pain (**b**). **c** Lateral view chest radiograph showing left pleural effusion and fullness of the anterior mediastinum. **d** Because the diagnosis was pulmonary embolism, a pulmonary arteriogram was performed. The catheter was in the pulmonary trunk. Selective injection at that level showed encasement of the right pulmonary artery (*arrows*). Note perfusion defects of both upper lobes compatible with the clinical diagnosis of pulmonary emboli. **e** Levophase of the pulmonary angiographic examination. Note opacification of the aorta (*A*). *Arrows* indicate meadiastinal mass extending beyond aortic knob. This finding is pathognomonic of a mediastinal tumor encasing the heart. At surgery, it proved to be a malignant mesenchymoma (or perhaps a malignant undifferentiated thymoma). Whenever we see a mass that extends cephalad and laterally from the aortic knob, the diagnosis of a mediastinal tumor should be considered. Echocardiography, contrast CT examination, MRI, and angiography can make the definitive diagnosis of pseudocardiomegaly due to a mediastinal tumor

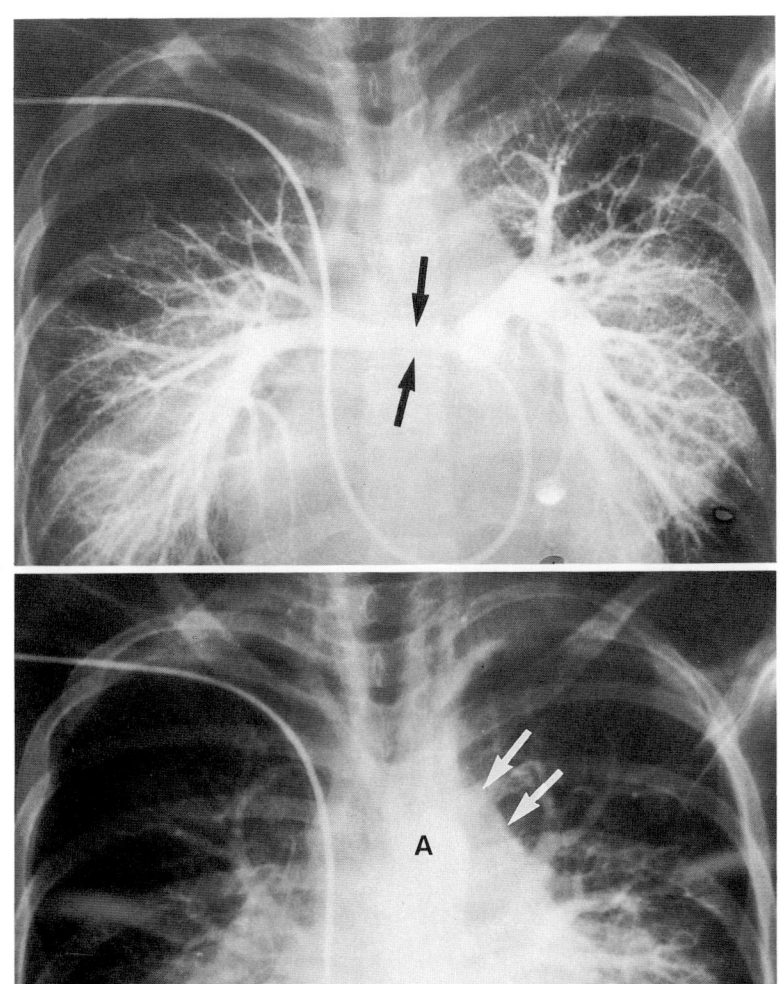

d

e

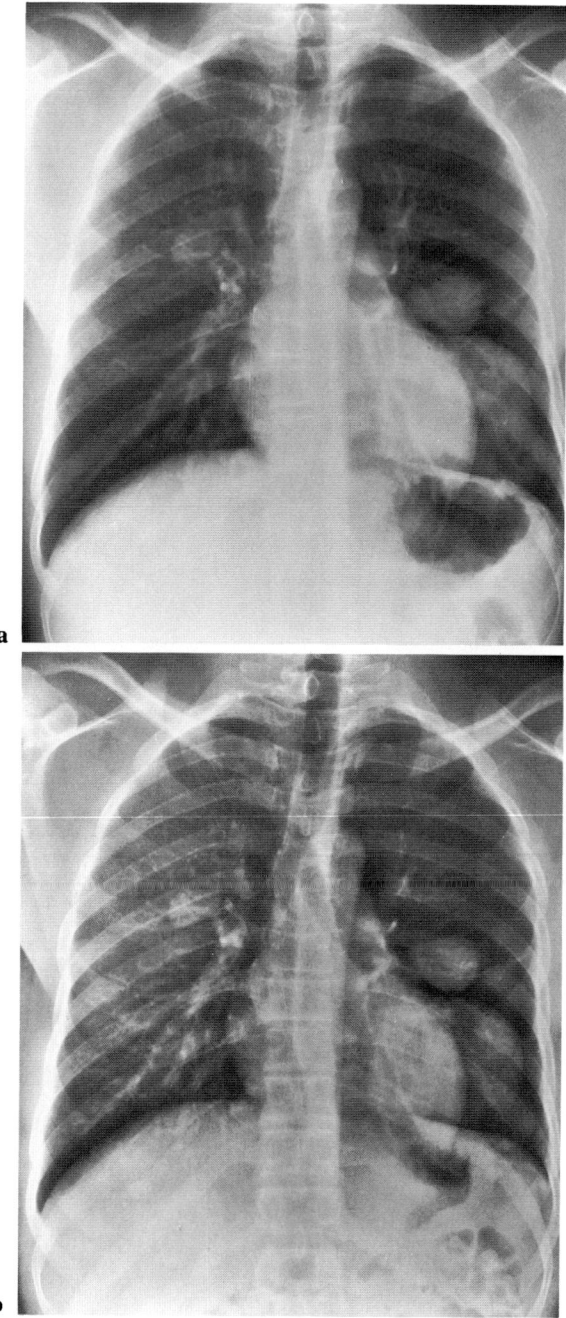

a

b

**Fig. 97a, b.** Value of AMBER study. **a** Conventional frontal view chest radiograph. Note bilateral pulmonary metastasis. **b** AMBER study showing to best advantage the metastatic deposits. One was seen through the diaphragm which was poorly visible in the conventional chest radiography

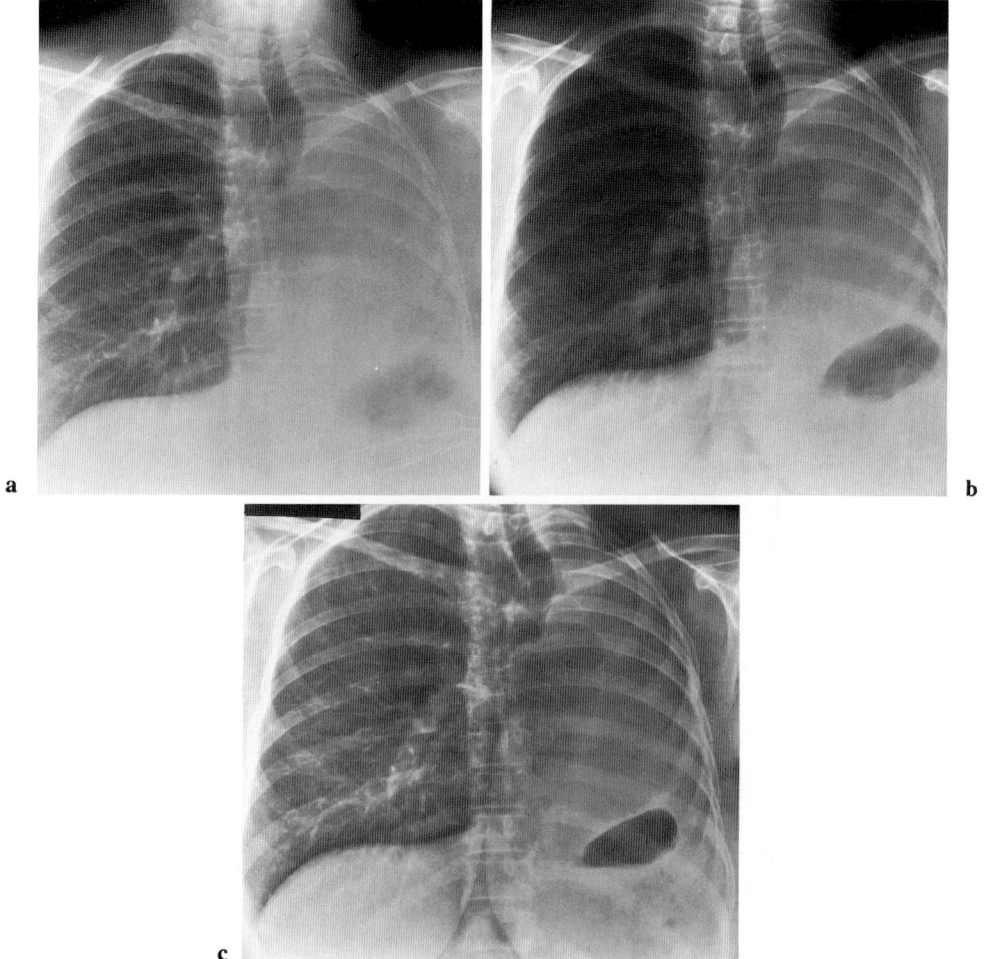

**Fig. 98a–c.** Value of AMBER study compared with conventional radiographs. **a** Frontal view chest radiograph exposed with lung detail. Note excellent detail of the right lung and poor demonstration of the pathology of the left hemithorax. **b** Overexposed frontal view chest radiograph which showed to best advantage the total volume loss of the left lung with an air collection in the mediastinum. Note that because of overexposure, the right lung detail was not well demonstrated. **c** AMBER study showing with excellent detail the right and left lungs

132

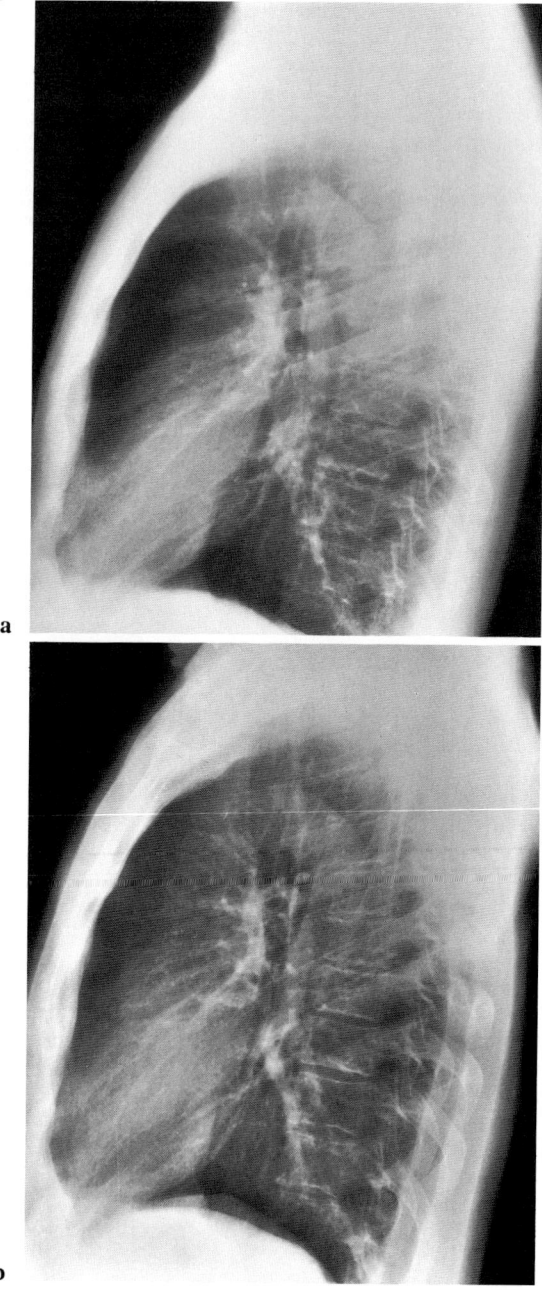

**Fig. 99a, b.** Value of AMBER study compared with lateral view chest radiograph. **a** Lateral view chest radiograph. The upper chest is underexposed and the proximal thoracic vertebral column is poorly defined. **b** AMBER examination showing with excellent detail the bony, pulmonary, and mediastinal structures

133

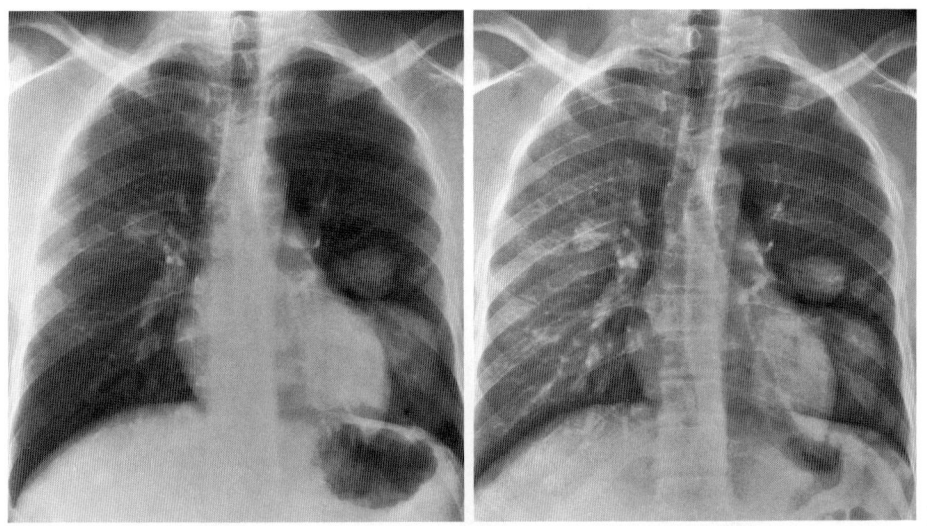

a                                                                                    b

**Fig. 100a, b.** Value of AMBER study. **a** Standard chest radiograph. **b** The same patient
as in **a**, but using the AMBER system. Note the superb spatial and contrast resolution.
(Photographs courtesy of J. Cullinan, Eastman Kodak Co., Rochester, NY)

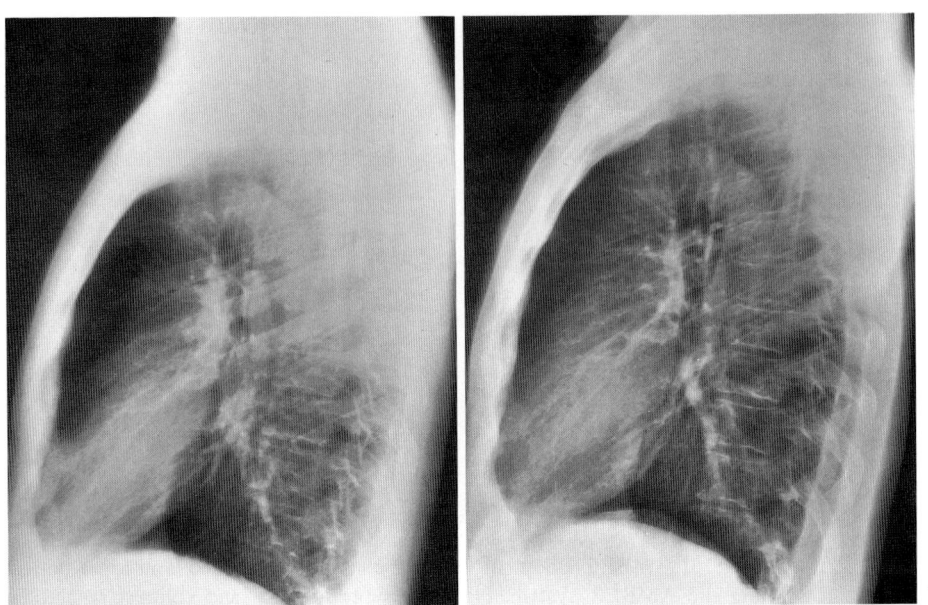

**Fig. 101a, b.** Value of AMBER study. **a** Standard lateral view chest radiograph. **b** The same patient as in **a**, but using the AMBER system. Note better demonstration of vascular markings and airways. (Photographs courtesy of J. Cullinan, Eastman Kodak Co., Rochester, NY)

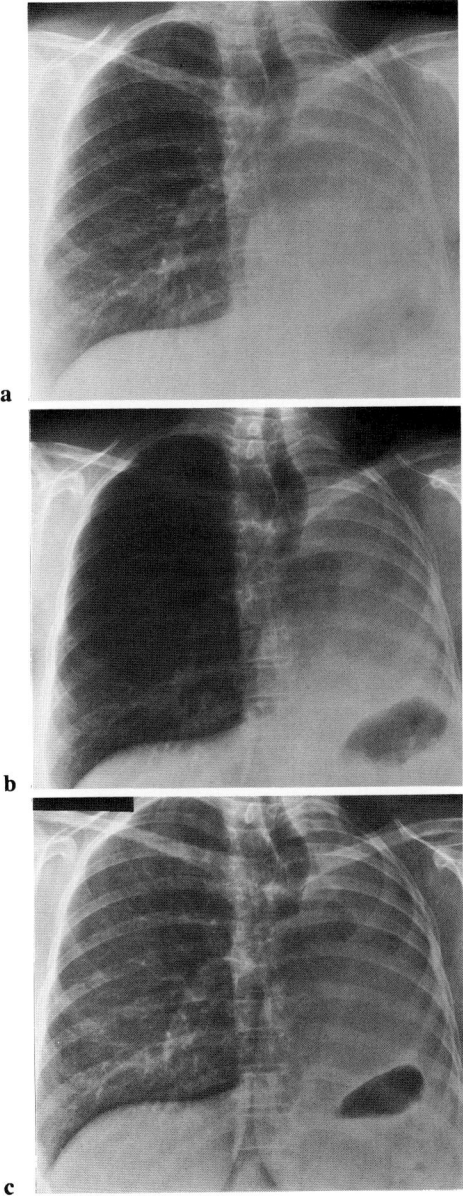

**Fig. 102a–c.** Value of AMBER study. **a** Standard frontal view radiograph using the lung technique. There is poor demonstration of the left hemithorax and agenesis of the left site of the lung. **b** The same patient as in **a**, but using the mediastinal technique for the frontal view chest radiograph. There is poor demonstration of the right side of the lung. **c** The same patient as in **a** and **b**, but using the AMBER system. There is superb demonstration of both sides of the lungs. Note herniation of the left side of the lung across the midline. (Photographs courtesy of J. Cullinan, Eastman Kodak Co., Rochester, NY)

**Y. Higashi,** Fukuoka University;
**A. Mizushima,** Kyushu University;
**H. Matsumoto,** Okinawa, Japan

# *Introduction to Abdominal Ultrasonography*

1990. Approx. 220 pp. 470 figs. Softcover DM 78,–
ISBN 3-540-51889-4

This book is designed specifically for residents in diagnostic radiology and those just beginning to undertake ultrasound diagnosis. Several features distinguish it from the monographs on ultrasound imaging of the abdomen that are already available.

The clinical chapters begin with a detailed anatomical description of the organ or system. The most common diseases of the upper abdomen are presented, with each entity completely presented on two facing pages. The clinical discussions are brief and clear; the high-quality ultrasonograms are accompanied by schematic drawings and body marks for orientation and better understanding. A variety of different probes are presented: linear, sector, convex and contact compound. Particularly difficult imaging, for example the tubular structures of the liver, is supplemented with color illustrations to portray the three-dimensional quality of the actual examination.

The book also includes short chapters on basic physics, equipment, scanning technique and a question and answer section at the end.

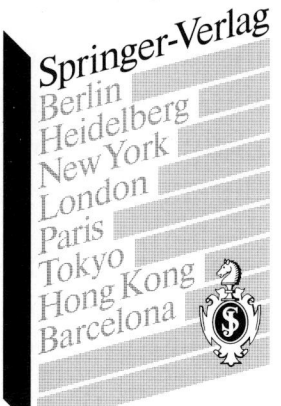

Springer-Verlag
Berlin
Heidelberg
New York
London
Paris
Tokyo
Hong Kong
Barcelona

**E. R. Heitzman,** State University of New York, Syracuse

# The Mediastinum

## Radiologic Correlations with Anatomy and Pathology

2nd, completely rev. ed. 1988. XIV, 355 pp.
302 figs. in 733 sep. illus. Hardcover DM 248,–
ISBN 3-540-18727-8

The second edition of **The Mediastinum** provides yet more complete coverage of the radiologic appearances of the normal and abnormal mediastinum. These appearances are correlated with underlying anatomic and pathologic specimens, permitting a better understanding of findings and more accurate diagnosis. The approach of the book is thorough, reviewing a wide range of abnormalities that the reader may encounter. In particular, this edition offers more precise insight into the radiographic appearance of thoracic disease. It also provides more extensive illustrations and an updated bibliography covering all literature since the first edition.

Prices are subject to change without notice.

Springer-Verlag
Berlin
Heidelberg
New York
London
Paris
Tokyo
Hong Kong
Barcelona